MISS-ING

MISS-ING

Psychoanalysis 2.0

Bruce Fink

AEON

First published in 2024 by
Aeon Books

Copyright © 2024 by Bruce Fink

The right of Bruce Fink to be identified as the author of this work has been asserted in accordance with §§ 77 and 78 of the Copyright Design and Patents Act 1988.

All rights reserved. No part of this publication may be reproduced, stored in a retrieval system, or transmitted, in any form or by any means, electronic, mechanical, photocopying, recording, or otherwise, without the prior written permission of the publisher.

British Library Cataloguing in Publication Data

A C.I.P. for this book is available from the British Library

ISBN-13: 978-1-80152-133-8

Typeset by Medlar Publishing Solutions Pvt Ltd, India

www.aeonbooks.co.uk

Human beings cannot help but consider themselves to be [...] missing something.

—Lacan, Seminar VI, p. 218.

I had always daydreamed about having a threesome with two women. I asked my college girlfriend how she would feel about inviting her sister to join us. She wasn't so sure at first, but eventually said she was willing and would ask her sister. Then, when she told me that her sister was also willing, I knew I'd never be able to do it. My manhood was in question. The whole fantasy came crashing down.

—An analysand

CONTENTS

PREFACE — xi

NOTE — xv

MIS-CONCEPTION(S)

CHAPTER 1
On the value of the Lacanian approach to analytic practice — 3

NEAR-MISS

CHAPTER 2
Transference revisited: how neurotic and psychotic patients use us differently — 41

MIS-READING

CHAPTER 3
The many faces of the imaginary — 77

MISS-ING YOU

CHAPTER 4
Love, warts and all — 103

MUTUAL MISSING (MIS[T] SEXUAL RELATIONSHIP)

CHAPTER 5
Notions of love in Lacan's later work   125

SOMETHING IS *a*-MISS

CHAPTER 6
Why people aren't what they seem to be, or what Freud teaches us about repression   143

CASE DIS-MISS(ED)

CHAPTER 7
The slings and arrows of outrageous fortune   165

MIS-TRANSLATIONS

CHAPTER 8
What makes translating Lacan's work so difficult   201

CHAPTER 9
Lacan in "translation"   217

MIS-SPEAKINGS

CHAPTER 10
The emphasis on the unconscious is back   237

CHAPTER 11
A Lacanian approach to Freud   255

CHAPTER 12
Why Freud? Why psychoanalysis?   263

MIS-CALCULATIONS

CHAPTER 13
Comments at the book launch for *A Clinical Introduction to Freud* (2017)   271

CHAPTER 14
Introduction to Seminar VI   277

CHAPTER 15
Brief remarks made at the 25th anniversary of *A Clinical Introduction to Lacanian Psychoanalysis*   281

MIS-LAID

CHAPTER 16
Review of Elisabeth Roudinesco's biography entitled
  Jacques Lacan (New York: Columbia University Press, 1997)   285

MIS-GUIDED

CHAPTER 17
A few notes on supervision   291

MI(S)-DIRE

CHAPTER 18
Afterthoughts: maxims and quotes   299

ENDNOTES   303

BIBLIOGRAPHY   319

REFERENCES   321

INDEX   327

PREFACE

Open almost any English dictionary and you'll find plenty of "misses" and "mis-es" relevant to psychoanalytic theory and practice:

> Misally (with the analysand against his/her parents, for example, or partner)
> Misappropriate (someone's words as if they were one's own, for instance)
> Misbehave (self-disclose, for one)
> Misdiagnose (an analysand)
> Mishear (something a patient says)
> Misinterpret (a slip of the tongue or a dream)
> Misplace (one's notes, one's datebook, or one's glasses)
> Mispronounce (someone's name)
> Misrecognize (a symptom, for instance)
> Misremember (a date or statement)
> Mistake (one person for another in the analysand's history)
> Mistime (an interpretation)
>
> Misedit (another's words)
> Misprint (a name or citation from a text)

Misquote (something someone said aloud or in print)
Misread (a handwritten note or a published text)
Mistranscribe (a Seminar or something an analysand says)
Mistranslate (a psychoanalytic text or something an analysand says in another tongue)

Misidentify (with someone in the patient's life)
Misinfer (that something someone says means X instead of Y)
Misnavigate (on the rough seas of an analysis)
Misperceive (what is going on in a treatment)
Misspeak (make a slip in asking a question or setting an appointment)
Missteer (a discussion)
Mistype (a note to an analysand)

Misadvise (a supervisee)
Misapply (psychoanalytic theory to the case at hand)
Misattribute (blame for a problem in the analysis to the analysand)
Mischaracterize (someone's complaint)
Misunderstand (the goals of analysis)

Miscalculate (how much the analysand owes)
Miscarry (by barking up the wrong tree)
Mischoose (one's words)
Misconceive (what is happening in the room)
Misconduct (the patient to the couch before she/he is ready)
Misconstrue (the purport of the analysand's words)
Misdirect (the treatment)
Misemploy (the session time)
Misfile (one patient's notes in another's file)
Misfire (by interpreting too soon)
Mishandle (a patient's gripe)
Misinform (a potential analysand about what to expect)
Mislay (the key to one's office)
Mislead (a potential analysand about how long the process is going to take)
Mismanage (the preliminary meetings by using the couch)
Mistreat (an analysand by acting peremptorily)
Mistrust (someone's story)

In short, misanalyze!

Analysts, being human, make mistakes just like everyone else. We often miss what we shouldn't miss, showing our *lack* of attention, foresight, acumen, dexterity, and flexibility. We even occasionally miss appointments (some analysts far more often than others)!

Certain psychoanalysts go missing in action, lapsing into inaction when they should be doing something. Others often miss something in a different sense of the term: miss their first supervisors, their old office, their early days when practice seemed simpler, their former patients.

To miss and lack is human, to fail to recognize one's failings disastrous!

One of my very first analysands, lamenting in a session her bad timing in the publishing of an article she had written on Bakhtin, came out with the graphic metaphor "near misses." Being attuned to different possible spellings of the latter sounds ("missus" and "missis"), I recalled that she had told me that she had fled her country of origin shortly after rejecting an unexpected and unwanted marriage proposal—that is, after having nearly become a Mrs. She didn't miss the connection when I slowly repeated "near … Mrs. … Jones" (a pseudonym). I never forgot the full-throated laughter to which that gave rise!

The reader will find in this collection many instances of misses, lacks, and failings in psychoanalytic theory, translation of analytic texts, and psychotherapeutic practice.

NOTE

All works are referred to here with the standard format of last name(s) of author(s), year of publication, and page number. Exceptions have been made, however, for (1) the *Standard Edition of the Complete Psychological Works of Sigmund Freud*, vols. I–XXIV (London: Hogarth Press, 1953–1974), referenced here simply by volume and page number (e.g., SE XIII, p. 23); and for (2) *The Seminar of Jacques Lacan*, not all volumes of which are available yet in either French or English. When available in print, they are referenced by Seminar and page number (e.g., Seminar XI, p. 23); when unpublished, they are referenced by Seminar and date of class (e.g., Seminar XIV, class given on November 11, 1966). I do not always adopt the translations given in the current English editions. A further exception has been made for (3) Lacan's *Écrits*, which is cited repeatedly. The page numbers given here refer to *Écrits: The First Complete Edition in English* (New York & London: W. W. Norton & Co., 2006).

A Bibliography of Lacan's Seminars and a References section are found at the end of the volume.

MIS-CONCEPTION(S)

CHAPTER 1

On the value of the Lacanian approach to analytic practice

(This paper initially appeared in *The International Journal of Psychoanalysis*, *100*(2) [May 9, 2019]: 315–332, and was subsequently translated into German and Spanish. My responses to the designated commentators, whose reactions can be found on pages 333–367 of the same issue, were printed on pages 368–376 and are included at the end of this chapter.)

Rachel Blass at *The International Journal of Psychoanalysis* kindly asked me to discuss, in the section of the journal entitled "Psychoanalytic Controversies," what is unique to the Lacanian approach to practice and its relevance to non-Lacanian analysts. A few preliminary comments about this twofold task seemed to me to be necessary:

1. There is no single Lacanian approach to psychoanalytic practice. There are many different Lacanian schools and they do not all emphasize the same facets or periods of Lacan's teaching, nor do they all always interpret his work in the same way. Like the writings of Freud and Melanie Klein, Lacan's work can be understood in a variety of ways, which entail different views of clinical practice. My own grasp of Lacanian theory is apparently thought by some in the Lacanian community (especially in France) to be overly direct, transparent, and

simplistic, leading me to make excessively practical recommendations as regards technique—in a word, as overly "American." This is, no doubt, at least partly because the French rarely make *any* recommendations whatsoever regarding technique in print, and generally only discuss case material in highly condensed and abstract terms that give readers little sense of how they actually practice.

2. For me to indicate what is distinctive about Lacan's approach implies contrasting it with how non-Lacanians practice, which assumes that I have extensive knowledge of other analytic schools—both their theoretical frameworks and approaches to practice. This would be to considerably overstate my familiarity with them. I have devoted the past forty years to grappling with and translating Lacan's often difficult work, and have only in the past two decades begun to try to familiarize myself with other schools of psychoanalytic thought. Those well-versed in the work of other theorists are thus likely to find my characterizations of them somewhat reductionistic.

   My knowledge of the work of other theorists comes from my admittedly limited reading; and my knowledge of what sort of practice their work leads to comes from three main sources: 1) clinical examples found in the literature; 2) what I have learned about clinicians' practice from the analysts I supervise (who tell me about how they themselves practice, but also about the approaches they learned in their training analyses, from their teachers, and from hearsay in their institutes); 3) what I hear from analysands who come to me after having worked with analysts who trained in other forms of psychoanalysis, these analysands often reporting to me—even verbatim at times—what their analysts said and did.

   I mention all of this because when, at conferences, I critique examples of what I consider to be problematic forms of practice that I have found in the literature (whether by Owen Renik, Thomas Ogden, Ralph Greenson, or Patrick Casement), I am often told that—regardless of their apparent stature and importance, at least when they were practicing—they are in no way representative of what goes on in the field and that no one practices that way *today*. And when I give examples communicated to me by my supervisees and analysands, I am almost invariably informed that what I am critiquing is not psychoanalysis at all, even though everything I cite comes directly from the mouths of psychoanalysts, and even though I myself believe I can see how the practices I am critiquing grow directly out of the theory of practice formulated by certain contemporary analytic writers.

Many of us would like to repudiate what we see as travesties committed in the name of psychoanalysis, but it seems to me that psychoanalysis is what is practiced by psychoanalysts every day in their consulting rooms, not merely what is attested to in the literature. Many practitioners fail, like Freud himself often did, to practice what they preach, but my sense is that certain practices today that are relatively new in the history of psychoanalysis grow quite directly out of current theories and thus should not be dismissed as mere failures to practice what is preached. It also seems to me that what is relayed in the literature should be viewed as presenting what at least some analysts take to be *ideal* approaches to practice, rather than as isolated and/or dubious experiments.

3. I will not talk in this paper about how Lacan himself reportedly practiced or was rumored to practice. Inventors in the area of psychoanalytic practice, like Freud and Lacan, tend to discover new practices by trial and error, even if it is at times to their patients' detriment. Such inventors tend to break all the rules in the attempt to discover new, useful techniques, and we know that Freud repeatedly tried everything which, in his *Papers on Technique*, he recommended we *not* do (see Fink, 2017). Like Freud, Lacan is rumored to have done myriad things one would have a hard time justifying in any sort of straightforward manner on the basis of his theoretical writings. Accounts by patients of their analyses with Freud suggest he sometimes continued, even in the 1920s and 1930s, to do all kinds of things he had cautioned against (giving advice; commenting on analysands' intelligence, the quality of their work in specific sessions, and the likelihood of their becoming good analysts; getting overly involved in their affairs regarding work and marriage; lending books to them; bringing them into one's own home and family life; etc.). And accounts by people of their analysis and/or supervision with Lacan run the gamut from glowing appraisals of his ability to listen and guide them in the development of their own style, to diatribes against ultrashort sessions. All such accounts should be taken with more than just a grain of salt, tendentious as they often are; in my view, they impugn the man more than the theory. A perfect harmony between theory and practice is an ideal some of us may strive for but which few, if any, achieve.[1]

* * *

That said, let me turn to what I, in my necessarily limited experience of the wide range of psychoanalytic approaches in the world today, consider to be the main differences between a Lacanian approach—my own, which is representative of at least a few Lacanian practitioners—and most if not all other current approaches.

Radically different approaches to treating neurosis and psychosis

> *It is hard to overlook the fact that the notion of the unconscious is in part based on slips of the tongue.*[2]
>
> —Lacan, *Seminar XXIII*, p. 97

Whereas much of the contemporary psychoanalytic world seems to have adopted an approach to treatment that is used interchangeably with both neurotics and psychotics, Lacanians work very differently with neurotics and psychotics. Moreover, whereas there appears to have been considerable blurring of the lines between neurosis and psychosis in many schools of psychoanalysis—as can be seen by the success of categories like "borderline personality disorder" and "narcissistic personality disorder,"[3] as well as by the often-heard notion that people can be psychotic at certain moments and neurotic at others—Lacanians continue to define and refine their definitions of neurosis and psychosis as distinct clinical structures, even attempting to discern a psychotic structure in certain people who have never shown any of the well-known florid symptoms of psychosis, such as hallucinations and delusions (Lacan sometimes referred to this as "prepsychosis" or "untriggered psychosis," and in more recent years it has become known as "ordinary psychosis" or "everyday psychosis"). Very briefly stated, neurotics are viewed as those with a fully functioning unconscious, a radical split between conscious and unconscious, and a strongly restrictive ego; psychotics, on the other hand, are viewed as those without a fully functioning unconscious, with no radical split between conscious and unconscious, and with an ego that may threaten to crumble at times. One very obvious consequence of the absence of a full-fledged unconscious is that psychotics generally do not get jokes, especially those that play on two different meanings of the same spoken word—for example, "whether" and "weather" (as an elderly park ranger once told me, "Seeing my success with the ladies, my friends told me I should be a meteorologist because I can always tell whether"), or a kidnapping and a kid napping—or of the same idiomatic expression (for example, "I didn't buy it," "He didn't come," "I just had to beat it," etc.).

Lacanians continue to encourage their neurotic analysands to recount, associate to, and interpret their dreams, daydreams, and fantasies with the rather traditional Freudian aim of locating unconscious wishes or desires in them that are at odds with, if not the exact opposite of, their conscious wishes. The goal in work with neurotics is thus to call into question the stories and rationalizations told by the analysand's conscious thinking self or ego, the ego being the very instance or agency in analysands that works so hard to know nothing about the "unseemly" desires and drives that inhabit them. Lacan went so far as to call the ego our "mental illness" (Seminar I, p. 16) owing to its will not to know.

In my experience commenting on cases presented by candidates and analysts at psychoanalytic institutes, the presenting clinicians are often unable to tell me whether their patient has ever made a slip of the tongue (much less one that was put to any productive use in the analytic work), a parapraxis, a deliberate play on words, a metaphor (or condensation), or an obvious displacement—in short, they often seem to pay no attention to the very things with which Freud taught us to detect the presence and activity of a full-fledged unconscious, as if the unconscious were no longer on their radar, or as if they believed that the only worthwhile access to the unconscious was via their own countertransference. Lacanians, on the other hand, generally have the exact opposite focus: they seek to detect the presence and activity of the unconscious in their patients' speech—that is, in what they say and how they say it (e.g., how they manage to say the exact opposite of what they meant to say, often without even realizing it; or come out with compromise speech formations, as when an analysand of mine referred to the anus as "an erroneous zone," instead of as "an erogenous zone," proceeded to remark that he had skipped over the "g" in "erogenous," and then unreflectively went on to relate what a friend had told him about the "male g-spot," bursting out laughing when I reiterated the "g").

Note that everything I shall propose here about Lacanian practice concerns analytic work with neurotics—that is, people with a functioning unconscious—not psychotics.[4]

Countertransference

Most Lacanians endorse Lacan's (*Écrits*, p. 183) definition of countertransference as "the sum total of the analyst's biases, passions, and difficulties, or even of his [or her] inadequate information, at any given moment in the dialectical process" of analysis.[5] This implies that they are far more likely to view countertransference as indicative of their own personality, hang-ups, and/or ignorance than as providing access to their patients' unconscious. They certainly do not see countertransference as the new "royal road to the unconscious," as it seems to be viewed by practitioners from a number of other schools.

No direct use is made by Lacanians of the analyst's reverie during sessions, of images or impressions the analyst forms of the patient's life that aren't substantiated in some way by what he or she says, or daydreams or thoughts that drift through the analyst's mind during sessions. The analyst's reverie is considered to concern the analyst and not to inform the analyst in any straightforward manner about what is going on for the analysand.

Although Lacanians do believe that analysands project things *onto* them—for example, imagining that they know things they do not know, judge negatively things they do not judge negatively, or feel things they do not currently feel—Lacanians do not believe that ideas or emotions can be directly "put into" them. Analysts may feel many things in and outside of sessions, but do not view them as having been transferred in some unmediated fashion, by some unknown transmission medium or mechanism, from analysand to analyst. The analyst is understood as playing the predominant part in what he or she thinks or feels and recognizes that not all analysts would think or feel the same things with the same patient—not because some are less "sensitive" or "attuned" but because they all have differing life experiences and would position themselves differently in the analysis. One analyst might begin to feel furious and believe his patient is putting anger into him, while in similar circumstances another analyst might not become angry at all; where, then, is the fury coming from?

Lacanians conceptualize our so-called intuition about what is going on for an analysand—what I have heard some American analysts call our "radar"—as the product of our own background, psychological makeup, training, reading, and knowledge of the analysand at hand conveyed by the content, tone, and rhythm of his or her speech.[6]

When an analyst feels stuck or frustrated with a patient, it is not viewed as the patient's doing—that is, as owing to the fact that the analysand is trying to frustrate him or repeating with him the way she frustrated her mother growing up, for example. Rather, it is presumed that the analyst has not adequately grasped the situation, has not properly conceptualized what is going on, has not found a way of helping the analysand along, and/or has incorrectly situated himself in the analysis—as someone who must have all the answers, for example, or who should be able to satisfy all of the analysand's demands and alleviate all of the analysand's anxieties.

In short, countertransference is viewed as something to be taken note of, explored in the analyst's own ongoing analysis and/or supervision, and as instructive to the analyst in his future positioning of himself in the analysis, but not as something to be communicated to the analysand. This constitutes what is perhaps one of the biggest differences in technique between a Lacanian approach to practice and that encouraged in many other schools today.[7]

Conceptualization of the role played by affects

We find in a Lacanian approach a different view of affect as it manifests itself in the analytic setting than that found in many other contemporary approaches. As in a Freudian vein, certain affects that arise fleetingly are viewed as potentially misleading owing to displacement. Just as Freud tells us, regarding affects in dreams, "we must allow for their intensity being increased owing to displacement" (SE V, p. 461) or "reduced to a level of indifference" (p. 467), and must allow for their being turned "into their opposite" (p. 471; love appearing as hatred, for example) or attached to other objects (making "false connections" with them), so too in sessions, affects manifest a certain plasticity, may be employed strategically (although not necessarily consciously), and may even be trumped up, possibly in view of evoking something in the analyst—whether that be anger, pity, love, or anxiety.

An analysand of mine once seemed to get very worked up suddenly after a somewhat long and productive session, and then fairly quickly commented that he figured I would soon be ending the session and pretended to get upset so that I would feel sorry for him and keep the session going a bit longer, even though there was nothing in particular he wished to add! Another analysand would sometimes cry to defer the moment in the session at which she would have to begin to talk and work. Shortly after noticing the pattern, she told me that she had been hoping I might just let her lie there without saying anything at all.

The widespread technique today of what I will (following Kristen Hennessy, personal communication) call "affect hunting"—wherein the clinician is constantly on the lookout for the slightest affect that is expressed in a session or may possibly be lurking in the background, attempting to elicit it with the stereotypical question, "How did that make you feel?"—plays little or no role in Lacanian work. Anything that elicits affect in the analysand is viewed by many contemporary practitioners (such as Patrick Casement) as the Holy Grail, whereas, in a more Freudian vein, to Lacanians the evoking of affect without connecting it up with thought amounts to nothing more than "libidinal discharge," which may feel good momentarily but accomplishes no actual work—it does not constitute a step forward. It is only when thought and affect are brought back together that repression can be overcome (see Fink, 2017, pp. 55–63).

From a Lacanian standpoint, since anxiety is, as Freud (SE XVI, pp. 403–404) said, "the universally current coinage [or universal currency] for which *any* affective impulse is or can be exchanged if the ideational content attached to it is subjected to repression," anxiety typically appears in the place of all kinds of other affects that might otherwise appear in the consulting room. One might then wonder why analysts-in-training are often told by their supervisors today that they are doing something wrong when the affect that manifests itself in sessions they conduct is anxiety.

As for affective states that seem more enduringly characteristic of patients, Lacan proposes that we view them in ways that are radically different from the ways they are generally viewed in other schools of psychoanalysis. Patients who present with so-called depression or sadness tend to be viewed today as suffering from intense feelings of loss, and this loss seems to be most generally conceptualized as having been brought on by some failure on the mother's (or parents') part to provide adequate love, care, and warmth to the patient as a child. Contemporary analysts thus often conceive of the analytic setting as one in which the analyst strives to hold and re-mother the patient, to give the patient the love, care, and warmth—this is often summed up with the technical-sounding term "mirroring"—he or she missed out on as a child. With the analyst serving the patient as a belatedly "good enough mother," the adult patient is thought by many to regress to infancy in the course of the analysis, and to experience a thoroughly new developmental process in which the analyst re-parents him, providing him with "corrective emotional experiences."

Nothing could be further from Lacan's view of sadness and depression—or, indeed, from his view of the analytic setting as a whole.

To Lacan, in the majority of cases of neurosis, these affects represent what he calls a "moral failing": the patient—while sensing, if not knowing full well, that he has a great deal to explore about his past and that there is a lot going on within himself that he is unaware of—refuses or fails to muster the courage to remember his dreams, free associate to them, recall his daydreams, slips, and fantasies—in a word, refuses to face up to things by genuinely engaging in the analysis. Instead, he adopts a cowardly stance, which is that of steering clear of the unconscious. Should he show up for his sessions, he assumes no responsibility for what happens in them, leaving it up to the analyst to take the lead and get the ball rolling, often in the hope that nothing will change, which will prove that psychoanalysis (like every other technique he has already tried) is powerless to change him and that he is thus a hopeless case, meaning there is no point in his even trying.

If the patient becomes "morose," it is, according to Lacan, because he refuses to confront the fact that relationships between the sexes are not what he grew up believing they were—perfect in every way, for example, at least if you meet the "right person"—and that love and sex are far more fraught and complicated than he wishes they would be, he being willing to accept only some sort of intense, romantic, and indeed fusional form of love (*l'amour fou*, or "crazy love" as Van Morrison called it, although he was hardly the first to do so) in which he can forget or lose himself altogether.[8] Nothing else will do.

If the patient feels "guilty," it is, in Lacan's view, because he refuses to reckon with the fact that he has "given up on his own desire," has allowed his own will to be eclipsed by others' wills, and is perhaps even getting a secondary gain from playing the martyr, feeling like the victim of others' bad behavior. He does not face up to the fact that, although there is no ultimate reason for *his* being in the world, for his desires or for his various satisfactions, others' desires and enjoyments are no more justified than his own and thus have no claim to be deferred to. This turns the more usual understanding of guilt on its head: guilt does not arise when I impulsively do something and then wish I had not; guilt arises when I shy away from doing what I really want to do.

In short, many of the affects for which patients are often excused and even pitied today by analysts, being theorized as arising from poor early parenting (of which there is plenty, I doubt anyone would argue with that), are viewed by Lacan as ethical stances adopted by patients with respect to knowledge, stances that generally entail a refusal to know about themselves, about the unconscious, and about the actual worlds of love and sex.

The implications of this radically different view are considerable as regards the analytic setting. For Lacanians, the psychoanalytic setting in work with neurotics is not a "holding environment," in the sense in which this Winnicottian expression is often used, not a cocoon or sacred space in which regression and reparenting occurs. Rather, it is a place in which the analysand is encouraged to work: to speak freely about everything, recount dreams and fantasies, associate to them, talk about the past and the earliest appearances of all of his or her symptoms, and so on (the analysand is encouraged to do so by the analyst in myriad ways in different cases, but most generally by asking open-ended, non-leading questions, leaving the analysand a great deal of latitude in how and where to begin, encouraging him to finish his sentences and stop censoring himself, not indulging his endless rehashing of everyday topics that have repeatedly led nowhere, and prompting him to do the lion's share of the interpreting himself). The past is considered to be of importance in its own right and no attempt is made to find or create some sort of link between the analyst and absolutely everything the patient discusses, as if the analyst had been there from the beginning in the patient's life and as if all roads in analysis led, not to the Rome of the patient's unconscious, but to the analyst. As in other approaches, "neutrality" is not taken to mean that the analyst is detached or uninvolved: his desire for the analysis to proceed and move forward is constantly at work. But he does not get personally involved in the analysand's daily struggles and life decisions, does not endeavor to become the center of the analysand's world, and does not use himself (his own reactions and reverie during sessions) as a major medium by which to *imagine* what is going on for the analysand.

For when we imagine what is going on for someone else, we do so on the basis of what we believe would be going on for us if we were in the same situation. If we imagine that the analysand must be devastated because he just got fired from his job or left by his partner, we may be surprised to hear that he was actually relieved, having believed that he deserved it, having hoped his boss or partner would finally take some action, and being overjoyed that he did not have to make a decision himself.

The analysand is not babied, and the analyst tries to avoid the trap of playing the role of a parent (Freud admitted that he fell into the trap of playing "too much the [role of the] father"; Kardiner, 1977, pp. 68–69). The analysand is given extra attention during periods of crisis, but this extra attention takes the form of additional sessions in which the analysand is still expected to work and for which he is expected to pay, not the form of endless unbilled phone calls, emails, texts, or other forms of contact. Rather than standing in for the mother or father (much less for "the combined parent"), the analyst stands in for or agrees to hold the place of the patient's unconscious; when the patient cannot figure out what a dream, fantasy, or symptom means, he often assumes the analyst knows its meaning and tries to get the analyst to provide it. The analyst willingly plays the part of the "subject supposed [that is, who is assumed or presumed] to know," the one in the room whom the patient *assumes* to have the knowledge of the why and wherefore of his actions, thoughts, feelings, and fantasies. The patient cannot initially find this knowledge in himself, as it is ciphered—that is, written in a disguised, displaced, or condensed manner in all the ways in which his unconscious manifests itself (dreams, slips, bungled actions, symptoms, etc.).

The analyst, for his part, knows full well that he does not know the why and wherefore of the analysand's actions, thoughts, feelings, fantasies, and symptoms. All he knows (like Socrates) is how to ask questions (see Fink, 2016, pp. 46–49) and hopefully how to decipher ciphered texts a bit better than the analysand does. Because the analyst agrees to be situated by the analysand in the place of knowledge (that is, as the one in the room who *must* know the answers), the analysand can have the necessary faith in the process to do the hard work of interpreting all of the manifestations of his unconscious himself—with the analyst's assistance, of course, above all in the form of questions and prompting.

The analytic setting is thus not one in which the patient's so-called needs are met or in which his demands are satisfied or given into by the analyst. Giving into requests and demands (whether for constantly changing session times so everything will be as convenient as possible for the patient, for hugs, for regular contact between sessions, and so on) generally leads not so much to satisfaction on the patient's part but to the multiplication of requests and demands—that is, to ever more of them.

An analysand, whose unusual work hours led to a great many sessions that his analyst agreed to reschedule, soon began asking for what essentially amounted to sessions on demand, requesting appointments that were convenient for him in that he was, at those times, finally awake and not drunk, high, or hung over. The times he requested became increasingly inconvenient for his analyst, who ended up constantly reworking her own schedule to accommodate him.

The goal in Lacanian work is to *defer* such requests and demands with a view to bringing out the desire that is hiding behind them or immanent in them. At the outset of an analysis, the patient's desire is usually covered over, unclear, tied in knots, and/or subjugated to the desires of those around him. The analyst does not give what he may have to give, whether that be warmth, sympathy, recommendations, advice, or obvious interpretations. Instead he gives what he does not have (which is how Lacan defines love—"giving what you don't have")[9]: he holds open a space characterized by a lack of knowledge, a lack of answers, and this spurs the patient on to find his own.

The analyst must not meet all demands for explanations and answers, but must keep open a space for lack—for not knowing, for a lack of satisfaction—for that is where the patient's desire can come to the fore. Whereas patients are often troubled by the fact that they do not know what they want when they first come to analysis, or want things that are patently impossible, their wants and desires become distilled out, decanted, and clarified as the analytic work unfolds, and they often leave with a sense of purpose and a determination to pursue what they want.

This brings us again to what might well be a fundamental difference in perspective between Lacanian psychoanalysis and many other contemporary forms of psychoanalysis, leading to a very different approach to practice. Speaking very broadly—too broadly no doubt—neurotic patients seem to be viewed by most analysts today as suffering from a lack of satisfaction. They are thought to have been deprived as children of their parents' presence, love, attention, caring, and warmth, and to be largely unable as adults to deal with loss or separation. Many analysts make a big to-do of the slightest interruption in the analysis initiated by the analyst—whether for vacation, professional meetings, family business, sickness, or holidays—as if they believe the majority of their patients can barely handle a separation of a few days, much less of a week or two (which might lead us to wonder, incidentally, how patients survived when American analysts back in the mid-twentieth century regularly took off the entire month of August, which French and other European analysts of all persuasions still regularly do today, sometimes even taking off both July and August!).

This belief seems so firmly rooted in analysts today that when their patients mention worries or concerns about what may happen to the analyst during such breaks, such obvious fears are rarely if ever considered to conceal wishes—as the most basic psychoanalytic theory would have us do (Freud, SE X, p. 180)—wishes that the analyst might fall ill or die in a plane crash so they would be rid of their annoying gadfly and be able to slide back into the restful forgetfulness of oblivion when it comes to the unconscious, for example! Nor are such worries read as suggesting that the patient feels his analyst to be an all-too-pressing and overwhelming presence in his life, a sort of "monkey on his back" who is breathing down his neck and leaving him no room in which to breathe easy.

Some readers may recall that Hillary Clinton once proudly announced that her daughter Chelsea, when asked at the age of four what gift she would like to give her mother, replied "life insurance," Hillary thinking it meant that "this tiny child wanted me to live forever." Had Hillary realized that it probably meant that Chelsea was unconsciously wishing her mother dead and was overcompensating for that wish by wanting to buy her life insurance, Hillary might not have so proudly proclaimed this to the world. As a small girl, Chelsea probably thought life insurance was something that would ensure that her mother stayed alive—in a word, Chelsea probably thought it was something that could protect her mother from Chelsea's own wishes that her mother die.[10] In any case, Chelsea *had* to have been thinking about her mother's death to be wanting to buy her life insurance, and I suspect there were few medical reasons to fear for Hillary's life back in 1984.

Just so, analysands' "concerns" about their analysts, when those analysts appear to be in good health, obviously suggest repressed aggressive wishes toward them. Yet they rarely seem to be read that way anymore! To my mind, it is often the case that it is the analysts who make a big deal out of short interruptions to the analysis who are *themselves* worried about their analysands (and thus harboring certain aggressive wishes toward them), not the other way around. Just as mothers who resent their children often inspire or incite so-called separation anxiety in their children (as when the latter are being sent to daycare or school for the first time)—the children putting on a show of anxiety or fear when the mother is about to leave but being fine with the other children and adults there five minutes after she has left—analysts sometimes evoke worries in their analysands that are not "home grown," so to speak.[11] It seems to me that such analysts are thus wanting to be loved by their patients and resent them when they feel their patients do not adequately return their love, after they themselves have, they believe, given so much to their patients. (Analysts manifest love to their patients by listening intently, remembering what is said, prompting, punctuating, and only occasionally interpreting; but seeking to be loved in return by their patients is a serious problem that I have discussed at length elsewhere [Fink, 2016]).

My sense is that analysts today tend to view a patient as a needy baby who can't get enough of their love and attention, instead of as someone who is suffering from an excess of satisfaction and is in need of separation, separation from the person or instance in his life that is leading to an overload of satisfaction, satisfaction that is, naturally, fraught, disguised, and experienced for the most part as pain or dissatisfaction. Lacan's view would, I think, be that our patients are not suffering from too little satisfaction, but rather from too much neurotic satisfaction; that our patients are not suffering from inadequate presence of a significant figure in their lives, but from an overbearing, inescapable presence. This is blatant when a fifty-year-old analysand tells us he talks on the phone with his mother for an hour every day and has since he left home for college, but it is true even when he has not spoken with his mother for years and speaks as though she has played no role whatsoever in his life for decades. For he continues to carry her around in his head and feel oppressed by her and everything she ever said she wanted from him and from life in general. It is obviously not by putting physical distance between ourselves and our families and homes that we separate. Something far more difficult and complicated is required, something which psychoanalysis alone can provide, in most cases, life experiences, meditation, and other mental and spiritual practices being powerless to bring about genuine separation from the weight of the Other with a capital O—that is, from the desires, demands, ideals, and values we feel have been foisted upon us by our families and by society at large.

Satisfaction, separation, and scansion

Symptoms provide satisfaction, as Freud taught us (SE XVI, pp. 365–366), but we experience the satisfaction we get from symptoms as anything but satisfaction: as anxiety, pain, humiliation, and so on. The goal in psychoanalysis is not to provide the patient with satisfactions of which we believe he has been deprived, but is, rather, to have an impact on the patient's pre-existing satisfactions that annoy him, that revolt him, and that he absolutely cannot experience as pleasure.

We offer him another satisfaction, a different satisfaction in analysis, the strange but often compelling if not exhilarating satisfaction of deciphering his life, dreams, fantasies, slips, and bungled actions. But we also help undo or alleviate certain symptoms.[12] If the patient is to get rid of or give up certain symptoms, he must renounce or separate from the satisfactions that come with them, and psychoanalysis cannot proceed without a sacrifice of satisfaction on the patient's part. The patient must separate from actual oppressive figures in his life, but also from internalized figures that are associated with his symptoms. And such separation is fostered by the technique Lacan devised known as "scansion," which he defined as making a *cut* or break in both the patient's speech and in the co-presence of the analyst and analysand, the analysand being abruptly ushered to the door—sometimes in midsentence, sometimes after having said something strikingly paradoxical, and often before he has said all that he was thinking of or intended to say on a particular subject or on other subjects that day.

This practice—which leads to holding sessions of variable length, which have often been pejoratively referred to as "short sessions" insofar as they may well last less time than whatever the "standard session length" is in the local psychoanalytic culture, whether that be thirty, forty, forty-five, fifty, or fifty-five minutes—is designed to slowly but surely separate the patient from numerous things: obsessively trying to make sense by laboriously unpacking absolutely everything he says and tying it up in a nice neat little package; constantly vacillating back and forth about every topic or potential decision he discusses; attempting to simply bask in the analyst's presence instead of working; always reaching the same conclusion or getting worked up about the exact same thing in sessions; getting off on blaming the mess in which he finds himself in life on everyone but himself; getting off instead on blaming himself for everything; and so on. In all of these we find a wish for some kind of wholeness, completeness, or perfection—total explanations, perfect harmony, and a situation without lack or loss in it. Yet an important part of psychoanalytic work involves the encounter with the "bedrock of castration," which we might characterize as follows in Lacan's terms:

1) The encounter with the fact that explanations can never be complete, for something is always left unaccounted for and there is always more that could be said
2) There is no such thing as perfect harmony between people, whether of the same or opposite sexes, there always being "a psychological phase-difference" between them (Freud, SE XXII, p. 134), they always being at cross purposes (Lacan, 1998, p. 78)
3) That no one has all the answers, and that no future outcome can be thoroughly predicted in advance—one simply has to choose and make the best of one's choices
4) That one cannot do or be everything in life—one's time on earth is limited as is one's energy and abilities.

Stated differently, coming to grips with castration means accepting and even embracing the fact that we are beings with serious limitations: limited intelligence, creativity, ability, time, energy, and so on. Castration means we are not whole, do not have everything we want, cannot be everything we might have wanted to be, cannot do everything we may have wanted to do. We are not omnipotent, omniscient, immortal beings.

One of my adult analysands concluded early in life that the only way to win his parents' love and esteem was to know everything for his father and be a muscle-bound athlete for his mother. Let me emphasize that this was *his* conclusion, *his* interpretation of his parents' desires and values, one that was not reached by his siblings. He undertook to learn everything in a certain domain—not with any particular goal in sight, not in view of doing anything with it, but just so he would never be caught out not knowing something he might be asked about it. He spent his time fantasizing that he had superpowers—which curiously aligns with the current obsession with magical powers in a Harry Potter-nourished culture (its roots obviously go back further, at least to *Superman*, *Bewitched*, *The Bionic Woman*, and so on)—which involved having extra standard deviations of IQ in addition to his considerable native intelligence. This would, he felt, place him off the charts, among the greatest geniuses of all time, and would ensure that he would invent something new and enduring that would put him on the map, inscribing him in history. And nothing else, no other form of work using his mind, seemed to him to be of any value whatsoever. With him, it was all or nothing: he had to "shoot the moon" (as in hearts, the card game, a risky endeavor that can fail catastrophically), otherwise there was no point in even trying.

In the realm of physical strength and athletic ability, he wanted to pump up and slim down, and spent years devising diets and exercise programs for himself, none of which he would actually execute until they were "optimal"—in other words, perfect, which nothing can ever be in any sort of absolute terms, even if plenty of diets and exercise regimes can be good for this or that purpose. He would occasionally embark upon one or another "kick," as we might call them, using this new approach or that, but he never stuck with anything and never pursued the more modest goal of simply trying to eat and exercise in such a way as to promote general health and vitality. The Eastern meditation and martial arts practices he engaged in for decades primarily fostered his belief that he could become superhuman, both mentally and physically.

It has only been in recent years, owing to his analysis, that he has stopped fantasizing about extra standard deviations of IQ and has even reckoned with the fact that he personally always preferred physical activity and labor to intellectual work. He realized he actually hated school and college, even though he always enjoyed contemplating life and figuring people out, and has begun to stop telling himself he has to do something exceptional that will make him go down in history. Although still conflicted about sports and muscle mass, he no longer feels the need to radically transform his body or break any speed records.

What did I do to foster these changes? I asked myriad questions, and the analysand, who was already prone to introspection, easily took up the project and began asking himself all kinds of questions. We explored his past in detail, including all those mornings when he had no desire to leave home and trudge off to class, and all the unpleasant experiences he had with teachers and professors. When the analysand would repeat assertions he had made his whole life about what he wanted and what he did not want, I would often punctuate those assertions with a monosyllabic "huh" or "hum," leaving it to him to decide whether I was calling them into question or affirming them, allowing him to project his own doubts and uncertainties onto my punctuations (see Fink, 2007, chapter 3). I would often underscore, as it were, parts of the assertions he made, such as "My mother wanted me to become a great writer," repeating back to him, "Your *mother* wanted you to," in order to encourage him to talk about what he himself wanted, insofar as it might be different from or diametrically opposed to what his mother wanted.

Our work together seems to have allowed him to begin the difficult process of accepting that he is who he is, with the limitations that he—like everyone else—has, and that this is good enough. The intense pleasure he formerly derived from simply fantasizing that he was someone else—Superman and Einstein all wrapped into one—which would then lead to intense dissatisfaction with his daily life, has abated and he now derives a certain amount of a different kind of satisfaction from what he actually does. The excessive neurotic satisfaction of fantasizing has been progressively pared away, given up, sacrificed—in a word, castrated—and other satisfactions are becoming obtainable.

Many contemporary clinicians would have immediately taxed this patient with narcissism, and he had, in fact, received the diagnosis of "narcissistic personality disorder" from previous therapists he had worked with. But I think it is plain that he retreated into fantasy because he felt worthless as he actually was, not because he truly had some grandiose sense of himself, and that those fantasies had to be gradually given up and replaced with something else. The fantasies had become more important to the patient than his own self and life; they had come to constitute a precious object (an ideal ego) that had to be renounced, sacrificed; he had to allow himself to be castrated of it. As he himself put it, he had to deal with the "forced choice," not of "your money or your life" (a choice which is "forced" because if you choose not to hand over your money, you lose it anyway along with your life), but "my fantasies or my life."

In short, he came to reckon with the fact that continuing to strive to gain the love and recognition that he had felt deprived of growing up—whether from the analyst or from other people around him—*could never make up* for the long-standing lack of these that he felt, but that he could derive a great deal of satisfaction from his actual life by giving up the incredible pleasure he got from fantasizing about being a superhero, a super-genius, or a super-playboy. He came to reckon with the fact that he needed to be castrated of or to castrate himself of such imaginary, neurotic satisfactions in order to move on in life.

Lacan explicitly relates the "scanding" or cutting of sessions by the analyst to the psychoanalytic notion of castration. Each scansion can be viewed as a kind of mini-castration, separating the patient from certain problematic or unwanted satisfactions, useless illusions fostered by ideals of all kinds that circulate in our culture, and conclusions of his own to which he clings to the detriment of his own life and well-being. In my experience, most patients take very well to the scansion of sessions; the few who take issue with it for a while are usually those who have previously worked with someone who always kept them at least forty-five minutes or even more than the officially designated time, talked and interpreted a lot, and had a tendency to pity and coddle them. Lacan goes so far, at one point, as to say that cutting sessions "is undoubtedly the [single] most effective mode of psychoanalytic interpretation" (Seminar VI, pp. 485–486).

Whatever cards a patient is dealt in life, he makes something of them, puts them in a certain order, and plays them in a certain way based on his own reading or interpretation of the situation (that is, of the desires of those around him, the apparent intentions of the world at large with regard to him, etc.). Like all readings, his is only partial and approximate, and his specific reading has led him to a dead end in life. Analysis requires that the patient reckon with the fact that this interpretation is arrived at by him and cleaved to by him for his own reasons—namely, that it is doing something for him, he is getting something out of it, deriving certain satisfactions from it (in the case I mentioned, imagining himself adored and recognized by both parents). Parts of his reading need to be reconsidered and revised in order for that dead end to be transformed into a through street. *It is not the parenting he received that needs to be redone; rather, it is his interpretation of it and the stance he adopted with respect to it that needs revamping.*

In order to encourage the analysand to revamp his stance, the analyst needs to strive to home in on it: on the part the analysand played in getting himself into the very predicament about which he has been complaining for as long as he can remember and against which his whole life has been a libidinally charged protest. This will most likely never change if it never comes into focus in the course of the analysis, which is what happens when the analyst himself views the analysand solely as a victim, a victim of poor parenting, unfortunate circumstances, and/or an underprivileged background—which all too plainly exist, but fail to explain everything and are generally unfruitful in helping the analysand move on in life.

The focus by Lacanians on castration-oriented work—prompting the analysand to give up old readings, and the fantasies, stances, and satisfactions that go with them—seems to me to be light years from the kind of work I hear about from analysts trained in other schools.

To mention but one example, an analyst who thought of a neurotic female patient of hers as having suffered great losses as a child and as insufficiently loved as an adult, agreed to provide her patient, at the latter's request, with a list of the main ideas and words from their many months of sessions together leading up to the analyst's summer vacation of a couple of weeks' duration. The analyst hesitated at first, but eventually spent many a long hour poring over her case notes while preparing a very extensive list of what she considered to be the main ideas and terms (or idiomatic expressions) in their work together, coming to view it in the end as a sort of labor of love. The patient clearly received it as a gift of love, realizing how much work and thought had gone into it.

We see here an example in which:

1) The patient is viewed as truly unable to make it through to the end of the analyst's vacation without something extra, a gift of love and care.
2) The patient's request is taken at face value, instead of being explored to see what sort of desire may be lurking behind it (for example, the desire to know exactly what the analyst thinks is most important, instead of the patient having to grapple with that herself, or the desire to receive an expression of love or concern from the analyst that clearly goes beyond the call of duty, that is, beyond what can be expected from the analyst as part of her paid, professional duties, her work on this list obviously having been unpaid).
3) The analyst gives what she has—ideas and phrases gleaned from the notes she took—rather than what she does not have, that is, her desire (desire being based on and fueled by lack, according to both Plato and Lacan) for the patient to decide what the *patient* thinks has been most important in their work together thus far and to try to take it further in the analyst's absence. It is quite possible that the patient would have preferred that her analyst decline her request (as Lacan puts it: "It is not always what people ask you for that is precisely what they desire you to give them"; Seminar XIII, class given on March 23, 1966), even at the time, and later came to regret she had found out so much about what her analyst thought important, as it made it more difficult for her to arrive at her own conclusions.

4) The analyst works much harder than the patient does, rather than the ball being put in the patient's court. Always a bad sign, in my view!

Some will want to object that this is not "real psychoanalysis," that no one does this sort of thing; and yet, as I said earlier, we should view psychoanalysis as what analysts actually do in the privacy of their consulting rooms. Moreover, it grows directly, in my view, out of the approach to analysis promoted by her training institute. It reflects, too, an at times implicit, at times explicit strategy on analysts' parts to become the center and focus of the analysand's entire life, such that all of the analysand's wants and satisfactions revolve around the analyst. Lacan, on the other hand, argues that:

> The subject's desire must not be guided toward our desire but toward [another person]. We help ripen the subject's desire for someone other than ourselves. We find ourselves in the paradoxical position of being desire's matchmakers, or its midwives—those who preside over its advent. (Seminar VI, p. 485)

Analysts from a number of persuasions might not take such a request on the patient's part at face value, preferring to interpret it on the basis of something that had just occurred in the session prior to the request being made, or on the basis of their view of the analysis as a whole (or of psychoanalysis in general). They might, for example, say something like:

1. "You have thought of a way for me to make up for the fact that I am leaving you; it would then be as if I were not leaving and then you would not have to hate me"
2. "You would like me to leave you with a list of important ideas so you can feed on them in my absence," or
3. "You think that if you can hold onto pieces of my mind while I am away, I will hold onto pieces of yours."

Rather than making comments of any such kind, Lacanians would instead, I believe, *encourage analysands to interpret their own requests* and why they came up at the specific moment in the work that they did, and would try not to ask leading questions that imply theoretical perspectives such as:

1. That analysands feel hatred toward their analysts when they go away on trips or vacation (as opposed to feeling something more nuanced and ambivalent, like abandoned and relieved simultaneously, for example)
2. That analysands come to analysts to be fed, whereas, in my thirty-seven years of practice, I have never heard patients talk about their sessions with me, as one apparently did with Winnicott, as "a good feed" (it seems to me that analysts "feed" such ideas to their patients far more often than the patients come up with such notions themselves)
3. That analysands believe that their analysts engage in similar activities and thought processes as they do, or at least can be induced to do so, which is a hypothesis that seems to derive directly from the imaginary register (in which I believe other people wish for and do things for exactly the same reasons as I think I myself do) and is based on the presumption on the analyst's part that some sort of "mirroring" or "empathic" process is going on.

Lacanians generally attempt to put as few words as possible in their analysands' mouths and to phrase the little they do say in such a way as to avoid bringing in theoretical perspectives. If our analysands end up formulating things in terms of hatred, feeding, and "transitivism" (as Lacan calls it, referring to what is at work when a small child sees another child fall down and the first child cries), better that it come spontaneously from them, and not from us, their analysts. If they end up describing their own experience in life and in analysis in Freudian, Bionian, Kleinian, or Lacanian terms, let it be because of their own reading and thinking, not because *we* have introduced such terms into our interpretations during sessions, rewriting their words with our own.

Focus on speech and nonsense

The focus in Lacanian work is not on constantly endeavoring to evoke or detect affect but, rather, on the unconscious as it manifests itself in speech. This speech, when we encourage the patient not to engage in "ego talk" but rather to free associate, is not necessarily understood by either the analysand or the analyst. Nor need it be!

The goal here is change as opposed to understanding, an emphasis on the latter (by the analyst, analysand, or both) proving at times to be an obstacle to change (see Fink, 2014a). The focus is not on the passage of some particular wish from the unconscious to the conscious, but to speech, whether that speech be comprehensible or not. This leads Lacanians to stress what is not understood—slips, slurred speech, non-meaning, and nonsense—rather than what is. Their concern is less with the intended content of what the patient says (the story or point the patient consciously wishes to convey) than with his actual utterances, which are often confusing, polyvalent, and overdetermined.

Use of the couch

Lacan's view of the analytic setting, which is so different from that found in many other contemporary forms of psychoanalysis, is reflected in a difference in technique as regards the use of the couch. Many analysts today seem to define analysis, that is, what counts for them as a "real analysis," as having a patient on the couch a certain number of times a week, usually at least four. This seems to me to confuse certain outer trappings of the setting with analysis itself, for one can practice supportive psychotherapy, CBT, mindfulness, coaching, or hypnotherapy under those exact same conditions, even if few people do. Analysts today very often ask patients who come seeking analysis—or whom they are able to talk into beginning psychoanalysis—to lie on the couch right from the outset. Freud himself often did this, but he tells us that he did so primarily because he could not stand to be looked at for eight or more hours a day (SE XII, p. 134), not because he felt it crucial and not because he thought everyone should do so, especially right from the first session.

Patients who are totally new to analysis, but who are directed to the couch immediately, often find it intolerable to begin to work with someone in such an unfamiliar way, feeling they need visual cues from their interlocutor before being able to go on with what they are saying, and before they are willing to reveal things that are difficult for them to discuss. They often end up *sitting* up on the couch instead of lying down, twisting around to look at the analyst, or requesting to move to the chair now and then; and this can lead to a confusing situation for both parties, wherein neither knows where in the room the analysand is going to be on any specific day.

Freud formulated the notion of the "preliminary meetings" (or "preliminary interviews," as they are sometimes called; SE XII, pp. 124–125) in which one tries to see if an analysis can, in fact, be undertaken between the two parties, is advisable, and under what conditions. Lacanians subscribe to the importance of preliminary meetings and recommend an often extended period of face-to-face meetings in which the analyst does not consider asking the patient to lie on the couch until such time as the patient has formulated for himself a question that can drive the analytic work, that can drive it in such a way that the patient no longer feels the need to keep asking the analyst to validate or confirm what he is saying, or to see if it is of interest to the analyst. It is becoming of interest to the patient—that is all that counts! He has developed an autonomous desire to explore his dreams, daydreams, and fantasies, and stops asking what the analyst wants him to talk about at each session. It is only once a patient becomes an analysand—that is, someone who does the analyzing himself—and begins to consistently pick up the thread from prior sessions and take up the exploration of his own psyche without constant help and/or approval from the analyst (whether in the form of verbal or visual encouragement) that he is directed to the couch.[13]

This puts the ball in the analysand's court—both the day's agenda and work come from the analysand, not the analyst, who merely assists in the process, hitting the ball back when it comes his way.

Not every neurotic patient will come to formulate a question of his own that can drive the analytic work, regardless of how much curiosity the analyst manifests by raising myriad questions, regardless of how much the analyst encourages him to wonder about significant events and turning points in his past, and regardless of how much latitude the analyst gives him to take the reins of the work. Such patients never truly become analysands, leave the curiosity and interpreting to the analyst, and remain libidinally attached to a lifelong complaint that, "through no doing of their own," things have not gone well for them. (Why, then, would we *ever* direct them to the couch?) We may at times feel we have failed the patient, as we have been unable to "kick start" his desire, so to speak—that is, spur him on to formulate a question capable of fueling the analytic work. Yet it is an open question whether anyone else would have been able to for that particular patient at that specific moment in time. Perhaps his time had simply not yet come, life not having led him to "a satisfaction crisis" (Fink, 1997, pp. 8–10) severe enough to make him truly open to the possibilities of psychoanalysis—that is, severe enough to outweigh the gains he derived from his symptoms, severe enough to force him beyond the natural human tendency (or even passion) we all share not to want to know anything about the workings of our own unconscious.

In conclusion

Lacan might be thought to provide a few useful techniques that virtually any analyst can add to his analytic toolbox. For example, punctuation and oracular interpretation (which I have barely touched on here)[14] may be more or less seamlessly added by some practitioners, and use of the couch may be delayed until such time as the patient has truly become an analysand. Other Lacanian techniques, such as scansion, would seem to require something of a paradigm shift. Like any other approach, Lacanian technique is integrally connected to Lacanian theory, and thus the degree to which other clinicians can and/or should attempt to incorporate such techniques into their practice depends on the degree to which they grasp and embrace the theory.[15]

Responses to commentators

I would like to thank my respondents for their thoughtful consideration of my work and for opening up possible avenues of fruitful dialogue between Lacanian and non-Lacanian approaches to psychoanalysis. Their responses suggest points of convergence as well as of divergence, points that would allow us—assuming we begin from detailed case material—to highlight how we would approach things similarly or differently, and how we would conceptualize what is going on with mutual respect for each other's thinking, even as we might nevertheless arrive at diametrically opposed conclusions and take different tacks in our analytic practice.

Certain of their responses also bring home to me once again the degree to which "the very foundation of interhuman discourse is misunderstanding" (Seminar III, p. 184). In the course of my paper (which was already twice as long as it was supposed to be), certain topics could only be touched upon briefly and the clinical vignettes I provided were necessarily condensed and incomplete. As we shall see, myriad misunderstandings revolve around the Lacanian technique of "scansion," which leads the analyst to conduct sessions of variable length; here once again, although I spoke very little in my paper about it (having discussed it at great length in print elsewhere; see, for example, Fink, 2007, chapter 4), it received the lion's share of my commentators' attention, just as it does when I present Lacan's work on just about any topic at non-Lacanian institutes around the world.

I will address the responses in the order that seems to me to make the most sense.

1) Alfred Margulies

Alfred Margulies' paper (*IJP*, 2019, pp. 341–351) warrants considerable commentary. Margulies seems to have concluded, on the basis of my discussion, that Lacanians simply dismiss out of hand affects that appear in the course of an analysis, whereas the point I tried to make is that we do not take them at face value. We try to discover whether, as Freud tells us regarding affects in dreams, "their intensity [has been] increased owing to displacement" or "reduced to a level of indifference," and must allow for their being turned "into their opposite" (SE V, pp. 461, 467, and 471). They are considered useful in grasping what is going on in the analytic setting, but not taken as transparently indicative of the analysand's Truth.

I would agree with Margulies that grief (specifically grief for the loss of a loved one) should not be understood in the same way as depression or guilt. I would nevertheless refer him to a passage found in Lacan's Seminar VIII, *Transference,* from a class given shortly after Lacan had lost his own father:

> Hasn't it ever struck you at some turning of the way that something was missing in what you gave to those closest to you? And not simply that something was missing, but that there was something that left the abovementioned loved ones irremediably missed by you? What could that be?
>
> Being an analyst allows you to understand it—with those close to you, you have merely revolved around the fantasy that you have basically sought to satisfy through them. This fantasy has more or less replaced them with its own images and colors.
>
> The being you can suddenly be reminded of by some accident, of which death is clearly the example that makes us best understand its full resonance, this veritable being—should you so much as call it to mind—flees and is already eternally lost. Yet it is this being that you are attempting to connect up with along the paths of your desire. But *this* being [*être-là*, which is also the French for *Dasein*] is yours. As analysts, you are well aware that it is, in some sense,

because you failed to want it that you also basically missed it. But at least here you are at the level of something that is your own fault, and your failure reflects the precise magnitude of that fault.

Is it because you made mere objects, so to speak, of these other people you have cared for so poorly? Would that you *had* treated them like objects, objects whose weight, taste, and substance we savor! Today you would be less troubled by your memories of them. You would have given them their due, paid them the proper homage and love. (pp. 36–37)

Perhaps even our grief for lost loved ones is not altogether what it seems to be at first glance …

Margulies seems to have misconstrued my comment about "visual cues." They are often considered by those new to the analytic situation (and to the population at large) to be essential to "understanding" their interlocutor; I have argued in many places (e.g., Fink, 2007, chapter 8; 2014a, chapter 5; 2014b, chapter 2) that body language is anything but transparently readable, being subject to different conventions in different cultures and locales (numerous books purport to explain how to read people from different cultures),[16] and that we often read it incorrectly, mostly seeing what we expect or want to see in others' faces, postures, and movements. I was certainly not saying that an analyst would obviously find visual cues of importance during the preliminary sessions and then reluctantly give them up when the analysand moves to the couch; rather, I was saying that when *patients* are immediately put on the couch, some of them find it difficult to give up cues that the patients are used to relying on (for better or for worse, for they are often mistaken as to their meaning) in everyday life.

Those new to analysis sometimes believe that their analysis will be successful if they just find the right analyst—that is, if there is the right "fit" between themselves and their analyst. This belief is usually based on little knowledge of the analytic process and grows, instead, out of the commonly heard view regarding love: all will be well when we find "the right person," as if there were one and only one person "out there" for us: "the One." Patients may well focus on the "singular presence," as Margulies calls it, of their analyst, and that may have something to do with their own desire and personality, but I would suggest that it is more often a product of the preconceptions and misconceptions about love that circulate in Western culture, and that are fostered by practitioners who dwell on the notion of "fit."

Margulies argues that the fact that the analyst "willingly play[s]" any part whatsoever "does not escape its own inevitable countertransferential problematics." Does he wish to suggest that the fact that the analyst sets himself aside and allows the patient to fill the sessions with his own thoughts, associations, feelings, fears, etc., for example, willingly playing thereby the role of listener, brings with it a problematic form of countertransference? The fact that we, as individuals, are drawn to and even train to fill such a role is something we all discuss in our training analyses; it seems to me that it only becomes problematic when we are so attached to thinking of ourselves as fundamentally good, special, understanding, and helpful people that anything in the analysis that suggests we are not gets in the way of our listening and remembering what is said. Playing the role of the listener may be characterized as implying countertransference, but it seems to me to play a very minor role in most cases.

Does the fact that a mechanic works on my car instead of his own, that an accountant does my taxes instead of his own, or that a hairdresser does his clients' hair instead of his own bring with it a problematic form of countertransference? Playing a role is as old as medicine itself, and Freud reminded us very early on that we are simply placeholders in the analytic process—anyone who would take the trouble to listen to patients as we do would find themselves the object of all kinds of transferences.

Regarding Margulies' critique of "oracular" interpretation, I would emphasize that the important point I believe Lacan was making was that the interpretation in question be readable in at least two different ways—as opposed to having one obvious meaning—*even as it grows directly out of the analysand's speech*. Thus I do not believe it bears much resemblance to the "analyst's reverie." In my work with a patient who had had a great deal of tsuris around toilet training, and discussed it off and on for years in analysis, when he complained that he felt he had nothing to give when he wrote or taught, I once proffered "You don't know shit" (an Americanism allowing for at least two meanings: "You don't know anything" and "You don't understand excrement"). It led to a great deal of laughter on his part and spurred on the work in subsequent sessions. It was hardly "oracular" in the sense of requiring a great deal of thought and/or projection on the analysand's part to be fathomed, but it played on two different meanings simultaneously.

I have the sense that Margulies has misunderstood my cursory discussion of psychosis here (I am perplexed by this since he obviously read my much longer discussion of it in my 2007 book *Fundamentals of Psychoanalytic Technique,* which he reviewed in *IJP* in 2014). I have never suggested that what I call a fully functioning unconscious "is operationalized by the ability to play with language, as in jokes," as Margulies puts it, but rather that the fact that someone does not get jokes that play on two different meanings of the same expression (e.g., the interpretation I mentioned in the previous paragraph) can be a useful sign to the clinician trying to make a rough and ready diagnosis.

I have argued (Fink, 1997, 2007, 2014a, 2014b) that psychotics do not enter into language in the same way as neurotics do. Psychotics do not have the "anchoring point" or "button tie" (*point de capiton*) that Lacan discusses at length in Seminar III, *The Psychoses,* and in *Écrits,* and it would seem that if this anchoring point is not instated prior to around the age of eight or nine, it most likely never will be. This hypothesis is at least in part corroborated by studies of language acquisition, where it seems that if a child is not exposed to a human language prior to eight or nine, he or she will most likely never learn to speak. This anchoring point is thus either instated or it is not (the knot is either "tied" or it is not), which means, in accordance with Lacanian theory, that one is either characterized by psychotic structure (if it is not instated) or one isn't (if it is instated). If one is characterized by psychotic structure, one may hear voices and form delusions at certain points in one's life but not at others, but, from a structural standpoint, this does not mean that one is psychotic at the former moments and not psychotic at the latter. The term "psychotic" thus designates a largely permanent condition, not a momentary state of mind. On the other hand, those characterized by "neurotic structure" never hallucinate, for example, except under very specific conditions of stress (while being tortured, for example, or in a concentration camp), prolonged sleep deprivation, and/or psychedelic drug use. (In Lacan's later work, psychotic structure is characterized differently, the imaginary, symbolic, and real not being tied together in psychosis, whereas they are in neurosis, but the notion that neurosis and psychosis are rather fixed structures beyond a certain age remains unchanged.)

One need not accept the theory that for neurotics language has an anchoring point, and thus the thesis that neurotics and psychotics enter into language differently; but if one does, one can regret (if one wishes) that psychotics can never become neurotics, but that does not stop it from being the case.

Margulies suggests that scansion leads the analyst himself to play the role of castrator, whereas according to Lacan it is speech itself—above all, in the specific, highly unusual speech situation constituted by the analytic setting—that brings on castration. As analysands, it is in confronting our own speech, rife as it is with ambiguities, contradictions, and rationalizations, that castration comes about in analysis. *The analyst's scansions serve the purpose of not allowing those ambiguities, contradictions, and rationalizations to be forgotten* by being buried under filler and instead to have their fullest possible impact on the analysand. The scansions highlight the fact that the speaker often does not know what he is saying, says something other than what he meant to say, if not the exact opposite, and is thus of two minds, divided from what he thinks of as "himself," split into conscious and unconscious. Isn't *that* the very substance of castration?

The focus on ambiguities, contradictions, and rationalizations can, perhaps, be a salutary counterweight to "enactments" (a term Margulies uses frequently but which is quite foreign to a Lacanian perspective, for Lacanians would argue against the existence of "projective identification" [see, for example, Fink, 2007, chapter 7]), "enactments" undoubtedly being to some degree inevitable. I do not see how anything I said could lead to the notion that the Lacanian analyst "arbitrate[s] the limits of the [patient's] possibilities," as Margulies claims. The Lacanian analyst highlights avowals and appraisals in the patient's speech of *his own* possibilities, abilities, failings, ambitions, lacunae, and so on, without in any way jumping to conclusions as to what the analysand may or may not be capable of accomplishing in or outside of the analysis. Although the patient may believe the analyst knows what he is about and what he is "worth" (situating the analyst as the "subject [who is] supposed to know, which the analyst knows he is not"; Seminar XIV, p. 412), the analyst realizes full well that he knows nothing of the sort and that it is, in any case, not his place to make judgements as to what the analysand is capable of in life.

2) Ricardo Bernardi and Beatriz de León

The commentary provided by Bernardi and León (*IJP*, 2019, pp. 333–340) abounds with useful suggestions regarding the initiation of dialogue between Lacanian and non-Lacanian approaches to psychoanalysis. I agree with them that such dialogue should begin from in-depth clinical material, which is not the kind I was able to provide in my short article, clinical material being the foundation for all psychoanalytic theorizing. I disagree with them that Lacan's work begins from abstract, philosophical considerations which do not grow out of extensive clinical experience; indeed, I would suggest that Lacan gravitated toward philosophy and structuralist linguistics and anthropology largely owing to his concrete experience working as a psychiatrist and then as a psychoanalyst.

The reading public may not be aware of the clinical, experiential bases of the lion's share of Lacan's work because emphasis has been laid in the majority of publications about him on his more theoretical thinking. But a familiarity with the entirety of his work and spoken seminars suggests that his interest in such abstract matters as cybernetics, topology, and logic grew out of his reflections on his own clinical practice, on that of his colleagues, and on the cases Freud wrote up. Let us recall for the record that Lacan more than once cited Freud's famous quip: "We must always be prepared to drop our conceptual framework if we feel we are in a position to replace it with something that more closely approximates to the unknown reality" (SE V, p. 610)—that is, that more closely approximates our patients' experience.

Few practicing Lacanians today provide extensive accounts of their clinical work with patients, but there are some exceptions (Baldwin, 2015; Fink, 2014a, 2014b; Gherovici, 2003; M. Miller, 2011; Pommier, 1996; Swales, 2012), and these accounts are, I believe, quite nuanced and cannot be characterized in the reductionistic way Bernardi and León characterized the analytic work that I very briefly described in my paper: "the analyst refused to satisfy his [patient's] demand, the patient's signifiers were put into play, allowing him to position himself as a subject of desire." My impression is that they are above all familiar with the Lacan of the 1950s and rely on accounts of Lacanian work as carried out by a small number of infamous analysts in the Paris of the 1990s, rather than on how the vast majority of Lacanians around the world practice today.

Bernardi and León have, for example, never heard of sessions "going overtime"—by which they presumably mean longer than the supposed standard session length practiced by non-Lacanian analysts in certain countries or cities, which varies from forty to forty-five minutes in much of France (Khoury, 2006) to fifty minutes in other parts of the world—whereas I myself and many of my colleagues regularly provide preliminary meetings that run over an hour, and certainly exceed some if not all of the aforementioned standard session lengths on a weekly if not on a daily basis. I know of few if any Lacanians in North America who regularly practice what Bernardi and León repeatedly refer to as "short sessions" (of just a few minutes in duration, presumably); instead they practice "scanded sessions" that may be shorter or longer than the standard in North America (and can anyone definitively tell me what that standard is? For it certainly does not seem to be the same for all mental health practitioners, if one judges by the fact that certain insurance companies in the U.S. have different billing codes for sessions lasting sixteen to thirty minutes, thirty-one to forty-five minutes, and forty-six to sixty minutes.). Lacanians are, moreover, just as attentive in my experience as other clinicians to risks of suicidality, the safety of patients and their families, and so on.

Lacan's personal practice was highly unconventional, at least as unconventional as Freud's or Winnicott's, but that does not mean that the majority of Lacanians today practice as Lacan reputedly did. Lacanians are generally committed to lifelong supervision and group discussion of their clinical work; this may not always involve the kind of pluralism that Bernardi and León advocate (and a great deal could be said about the relative advantages and disadvantages of pluralism, but I do not believe this is the place to do so), but it does encourage analysts to consider the perspectives of those with different clinical backgrounds and sensibilities, and thus to regularly call into question their conceptualization of the cases they are treating. This is the kind of work that generally goes on in clinics, hospitals, and daylong or weekend-long seminars in which cases are presented and discussed in great detail. It is unfortunate that little of this makes it into print, especially in English translation.

I do not believe I have ever suggested that the analyst's countertransference should be ruled out as "a clue or indicator of the analyst's unconscious emotional response to his or her patient"; indeed in many places in my work I have recommended that the analyst pay close attention to his or her countertransference and bring it to his or her own personal analysis and/or ongoing supervision (see, for example, Fink, 2007, chapter 7). What I *have* said is that Lacan recommends that the analyst's countertransference not be revealed directly to the analysand and that it should not be thought to give *transparent* clues about what is going on for the analysand—that is, about the analysand's unconscious. For the analyst's countertransference may have far more to do with the analyst than with the analysand, not all analysts being likely to react to a specific patient in the same way.

Nor do I believe I have ever said that affects "are always misleading." (I wrote here: "As in a Freudian vein, certain affects that arise fleetingly are viewed [by Lacanians] as *potentially* misleading owing to displacement.") Working through affects related to loss and failure seems to me to be a part of virtually every analysis. I find it hard to locate any evidence of my ever having said that "oracular interpretation must be unexpected, gratuitous, playful, almost a joke," or of Lacan having ever said that. Interpretations may, at times, be playful (as in the example I gave earlier), and should certainly not be predictable, but I would hardly characterize them as "gratuitous" or as always taking the form of virtual "jokes"; they are, I believe, characterized as oracular by Lacan because they allow for multiple readings and put the analysand to work as he attempts to wrap his head around them. In the best of cases, they are *pithy and polyvalent*.

3) Lionel Bailly

To Lionel Bailly's very kind paper (*IJP*, 2019, pp. 362–367), I can only say "Thanks!" I fully agree with him that it is important that analysands not come to feel that the variation in session length means that the analyst is allowed to make up his own rules as he goes along. It should be made clear to analysands that the analyst strives to follow strict guidelines in scanding sessions—i.e., that he, too, is subject to the law and that his scansions are not made at random but obey a specifiable logic.[17]

4) Sara Flanders

Flanders' commentary (*IJP*, 2019, pp. 352–361) reminds me again of the gulf that separates Lacanian and non-Lacanian analysts' conceptions of neurosis, when she characterizes the neurotic's ego as

> susceptible to crumbling under the pressure of drives, or terrors of invasion, or burdens of grief, or the overwhelming by trauma. Indeed, the adolescent ego which often resorts to psychotic functioning, under pressures of radical change in the reality of the body, the increased power of the drives, the violent upsurges of unconscious material, stands precariously on the edge of these differences.

Either we work with totally different patient populations, are simply not talking about the same kinds of patients, diagnostically speaking, when we use the term "neurosis," or our ways of viewing what is going on in analysis are so far apart as to lead to what the French call a *"dialogue de sourds"* ("dialogue of the deaf")—in English we might say that we simply do not speak the same language.

Scansion is described by Flanders as reflecting Lacan's (and by extension the Lacanian analyst's) "frustrated countertransference," the analyst wanting more to happen in the session and discharging his "irritation" by ending the session when "the analyst judges the work not good enough." I cannot help but wonder where such a notion was gleaned from! I suspect that many analysts would be happy to stop sessions when they feel they have become boring, but I have never heard Lacan's variable-length session characterized in such a way; rather, sessions are generally put an end to when the analysand has said something strikingly paradoxical or contradictory, has raised a relevant question, or has most fully and forcefully expressed an idea (often one that is highly charged affectively) that much of the session seemed to be leading up to. Which is a horse of a different color!

My sense is that analysts who never underwent an analysis in which scansion was used have a tendency to project onto scansion a function that they themselves might relish: that of conveying to the patient that what he is doing is not good enough or is boring. Patients who have been in analyses in which scansion *was* employed will generally tell you that it operates quite differently, emphasizing points that are significant and likely to move the analytic work forward. In my own analysis, and in my thirty-seven years of analytic practice, I have seen few analysands who have objected to the use of scansion and the vast majority have found it to be a very helpful technique (a few have found it punitive, especially early on in their work with me, but they were generally people who found virtually everything punitive, including scheduling, payment, reiteration of their own words, and interpretations of all kinds). Although non-Lacanian analysts seem to be quite horrified by scansion, most patients—and I hardly think they can all be fairly characterized as fundamentally masochistic—appreciate and at times even enjoy it.

I find it hard to agree with the author that the practice of the "standard-length session" implies that "every session comes to an agreed-upon end." In my thirty years' supervising analysts, psychologists, and psychiatrists, I have very often heard about patients who continue to talk long after the clinician has indicated that their time is up, who refuse to leave the couch, or who keep talking nonstop out into the hallway or waiting room. It is not because a patient tacitly or even explicitly agrees at the outset of an analysis to having fifty-minute sessions five times a week that he is perfectly happy to stop talking when the minute hand strikes fifty. Plenty of patients complain bitterly about being stopped mid-sentence or mid-thought by their analysts, and feel rigorous adherence to the fifty-minute hour to be sadistic on their analysts' parts. I would point out that, in my experience, most analysts spontaneously vary session length by a minute or two, or possibly even three or four, precisely for that reason, which means that *the vast majority of analysts provide variable-length sessions unbeknownst to themselves*, or at least in a way that has, to the best of my knowledge, never been avowed or theorized in the literature.

It is well known that Freud himself did not religiously adhere to a fixed session length, even if he did generally schedule by the hour; he indicated that

> One occasionally comes across patients to whom one must give more than the average time of one hour a day, because the best part of an hour is gone before they begin to open up and to become communicative at all. (SE XII, pp. 127–128)

And patient accounts indicate that neither Freud nor Winnicott rigidly adhered to a fixed session length (see, for example, Little, 1990); consider Ralph Greenson, who sometimes held four-hour sessions with Marilyn Monroe (Spoto, 1993). If sessions can justifiably be varied in the direction of going longer than the standard time—which might, in contemporary parlance, be referred to as "a violation of the frame"—why is it anathema for them to be varied in the other direction? If the frame is sacrosanct, then all "frame violations" are presumably sanctionable.[18]

If it is a legitimate move to analyze the countertransference involved in practicing a fixed-length session as opposed to a variable-length one (and I am not saying that it is, but Flanders does it), why wouldn't we take seriously Winnicott's (1958a, p. 285) claim that ending sessions after a fixed length of time is an expression of hatred on the analyst's part? And what would stop us from contrasting that with the joy the Lacanian analyst experiences upon scanding a session when the analysand provides the fullest, most enthusiastic expression of a new point of view?

Lacanians do not tell non-Lacanians they *must* practice the variable-length session. Why can't Lacanians and non-Lacanians be viewed as practicing in equally legitimate ways, albeit with different rationales? Perhaps, then, we could focus discussion on other points of convergence and divergence.

NEAR-MISS

CHAPTER 2

Transference revisited: how neurotic and psychotic patients use us differently

(This paper was to have been given on October 29, 2022, at the Center for Modern Psychoanalytic Studies, at the invitation of William Hurst.)

I will start by very briefly discussing Freud's and Lacan's notions of transference, which concern only neurotics, for neither Freud nor Lacan believed that transference with psychotics was possible. I examined their viewpoints at length in my book *Fundamentals of Psychoanalytic Technique*, in a chapter entitled "Handling Transference and Countertransference." It turned out to be the longest chapter in the book, as there was a great deal of material to cover and my sense was that many analysts today no longer know how transference was defined by Freud or how it was understood during the first fifty years of psychoanalytic practice, it having turned into a term that is used to mean something quite different from what it initially signified.

That is an interesting topic in and of itself regarding the history of psychoanalysis, as the same could be said of many psychoanalytic concepts, like those of the unconscious and the drives. We might wonder why such concepts seem so subject to continental drift, as it were, and, to change metaphors, to becoming watered down. Lacan once commented that "Everyone knows how easily we forget everything that has to do with the unconscious" (Seminar VI, p. 60), and I suspect his comment might well be relevant here!"

The main characteristics of transference in neurosis

Freud's German term usually rendered as "transference," *Übertragung*, is a highly polyvalent word, whose meanings in various contexts (linguistic, financial, and others) include translation, transposition, transfer, broadcast, assignment, rendering, conveyance, transmitting, and bringing forward. Many of its meanings imply that something is conveyed or transmitted from point A to point B, generally speaking from the past, from some past relationship or situation, to the present, to the current relationship or situation with the analyst; something is translated from one language into another, from one context into another. The analyst may become associated with a specific figure from the analysand's past, or a whole series of figures, based on a wide variety of features, including:

- Imaginary: the analyst visually resembles someone from the analysand's past, perhaps even in just one tiny respect (which may be a projection, as it is later no longer even noticed by the patient)
- Symbolic: the analyst has a certain social position, background, or education like someone from the analysand's past, or uses certain words or expressions they used
- Real: the analyst's voice or gaze resembles that of someone from the analysand's past, his or her stomach occasionally grumbles like someone from his past.

Conflicts with those figures from the past are said, by Freud, to be reproduced or repeated with the analyst owing to the supposed resemblance. That brings them up for discussion in the analysis and the analyst strives to trace them back to their sources and get the analysand to discuss those conflicts in the fullest detail possible. For Freud, repetition is at the very crux of transference. Without that repetition, the analysand might never recall such conflictual situations from the past. For example, in everyday discussions with one's friends, childhood scenes and traumas may rarely rise to consciousness. With the analyst who strives to be a blank slate to the highest degree possible, they often do.

Yet transference concerns not just the analyst, but the entire analytic situation, including scheduled times, offices or virtual meeting places, couches, armchairs, noises heard in adjoining rooms, the exchange of money, etc. All of these can bring to mind forgotten or almost forgotten scenes from the past.

In contemporary discourse, however, transference is virtually only thought of as involving the patient's affect or feelings toward the analyst. As David Huntingford Malan (1995, p. 21) put it, "the word has gradually become more loosely used for *any* feelings that the patient may have about the therapist." That obviously then includes feelings that are *not* transposed onto the analyst from prior figures or repeated from the past, feelings that thus ostensibly arise from how the analysand experiences the analyst him- or herself as a person (like anyone else). You can see how far from Freud's initial definition this loose usage is.

Lacan's major early contribution to the study of transference was the notion that transference love grows out of the presumption that the analyst knows something of very great importance to the analysand, that the analyst knows what makes him tick and how to change what makes him tick. To the analysand's mind, the analyst is a "subject-supposed-to-know," someone who presumably knows what is unconscious in patients, to have special insight into what the analysand is trying to discover about himself. This is what leads, in part, the patient to project his own not yet conscious thoughts, thoughts which he wishes didn't exist, and which he is as yet unwilling to admit to having or unwilling to accept, onto the analyst. Hence the frequency, in our work with neurotics, of patients making comments to us like "You must be thinking I'm lying," "You probably think I'm an idiot," or "I'm sure you find me a horrible person," when that is quite clearly what the analysand is thinking about herself or when that is clearly what the analysand believed one or both of her parents thought of her or often said about her. The analyst as subject-supposed-to-know is thus clearly a stand-in or placeholder for the analysand's unconscious.[1]

We find here a clear divide between neurosis and psychosis as regards knowledge:

- The neurotic is someone who is bothered by knowledge (Seminar XVI, p. 303) about himself that seems to be unavailable to him, bothered by things of which he at least dimly senses he is unaware. He feels opaque to himself. He may have a conscious discourse about

why he is doing what he is doing and feeling what he is feeling, but senses that it is not the whole story.
- The psychotic, on the contrary, generally believes he knows all about himself. To his mind, there is nothing opaque *within himself* and thus the analyst is *not* a subject-supposed-to-know for him, certainly not someone who knows him better than he knows himself, certainly not someone who has special insight into the secret reasons why he is doing what he is doing and feeling what he is feeling. If and when something enigmatic does appear in his world, it is situated outside himself, not inside. Something is wrong with the world, not with something deep within.

My neurotic patients occasionally comment that I seem to know what they have said about their past and what they have told me about themselves in the course of the analysis better than they themselves do. I don't believe this has ever happened with any of my psychotic patients! They tend to insist, on the contrary, that they know exactly what they've told me and that I am simply mistaken for understanding what they said differently than they did, or for believing they've told me something they don't agree they told me.

Insofar as Lacan is right in thinking that transference love grows out of a presumption that the analyst has knowledge that the patient would like to have about what makes him tick, we have here a first obstacle to transference in work with psychotics. And insofar as Freud is right in thinking that transference involves the repetition of an earlier situation, and insofar as repetition is at least partially based on symbolic coordinates—in short, coordinates involving language and speech—psychotics do not repeat things with the analyst in the same way as neurotics do. For virtually everyone has noticed that psychotics do not use language or speak in the same way as neurotics do. The analysand who shows up at your office at seven in the evening instead of three in the afternoon and can associate to seven as the time at which one of her parents was officially declared dead is obviously neurotic, situating her "mistake" as a true bungled action that is of significance owing to the context and point in the analysis at which it occurred. We might fruitfully ask her if she is wanting to talk about that death? Or even wanting to find the analyst dead upon her arrival? With neurotics, such bundled actions tend to open up multiple associative doors.

The analysand who shows up at your office at seven in the evening instead of at three in the afternoon and can say nothing about it other than that she was sure it was seven or that *you* must be mistaken may not be repeating anything: in certain cases, a pipe is just a pipe and a mistake is just a mistake. There is nothing to analyze there.

The kinds of relations with prior figures in their lives psychotics repeat tend to be massive: we analysts are just like those prior figures, trying to exploit or persecute them just like the earlier ones did. Neurotics' repetition of relations with prior figures in their lives tends to be selective, taking up now one, now another facet of those relations, now one, now another detail about the analyst, too.

Like Freud, Lacan did not recommend deliberately trying with neurotics to bring everything into the transference or make everything happen through the transference. For Lacan, like Freud, transference is an inevitable part of the analytic situation, but its strongest manifestations suggest that something has gone wrong, not right, and that the analyst has not managed to situate him- or herself properly in the analysis. Especially early on in his work (1950s), Lacan talks (like Freud did in the Rat Man case) of transferences in the plural—that is, momentary projections by one and the same patient onto the analyst of figures and relationships with them from the patient's past, even his recent past. Lacan thinks of these as momentary obstacles or turning points in the "dialectical process" or unfolding of the analysis, not as something to be celebrated as indicative of some kind of progress. The main goal for both Freud and Lacan is to bring out a maximum amount of the material via memory and speech, and a minimum of the material via acting out and transferences.[2]

Historical perspectives on working with psychotics

Freud expressed the belief (around 1907) that psychosis involves the withdrawal of libido into oneself, into the ego—leading to what he called "narcissism"—making it such that the psychotic's libido cannot find an object or attach itself to an object. He therefore concluded that there can be no attachment on the psychotic's part to the analyst.

Theoretically speaking, we might postulate that a strong object cathexis usually stems from having lost an object—most generally speaking, the mother as the object of our first satisfactions—and that it would therefore seem that psychotics have never been forced to give up an object in the same way as neurotics have. You have to have been required to lose or forego it in order to crave it forever thereafter. (Lacan refers to this as the "extraction of object *a*.") We could thus wonder whether we should talk about a "withdrawal" of libido from an object or rather *a lack of object cathexis from the outset in the psychotic's life.* (At least two different possibilities present themselves here: the bond with the mother was never very strong to begin with, such that giving her up didn't lead to fixation on a lost object connected to her; or the bond was so strong that it was never or can never be broken.)

Federn was perhaps the first analyst to deliberately try to cultivate a positive object-relation with patients, sometimes by giving them chocolates, by talking only about pleasant things with them, and even by taking them to live in his own home (Maleval, 2000, pp. 350–354). This kind of object-relation remained at the idealizing level: the patient took the analyst as a generous helper or support of some kind, and possibly as a good person to imitate. We might wonder whether it makes sense to refer to this as transference at all; perhaps it would make more sense to simply call it "positive regard" or a "good rapport." In any case, it seems based on idealization—on patients being able to find the analyst to be some kind of ideal figure in their lives.

Henry Stack Sullivan, D. M. Mullard, Frieda Fromm-Reichmann, Harold Searles, and others, and then the Kleinians more generally, also experimented with the stance they adopted with psychotics (Maleval, 2000, pp. 355–359). Since the 1950s, most analysts have come to agree that psychotics *can* form attachments to the analyst, but they tend to be massive, often involving a total merging or confusion of self and other (relations known in French as *fusionnelles*, fusional), and potentially swinging violently from love to hate.[3]

Lacan tended to agree with these perspectives, viewing psychosis as involving two somewhat unique configurations of libido when that libido is invested in others, even if not to a very high degree:

1) It takes the other person as an ideal figure to be admired, imitated, or perhaps even absorbed into oneself.
2) It takes the other person as a persecutor or as the object of what he called "mortifying erotomania" (Lacan, 2001, p. 217). Psychotics may well experience themselves as subject to exploitation by an evil-intentioned analyst. We might understand this in some sense as "the reproduction of an earlier situation," insofar as one or both parents

seemed to have evil or exploitative intentions starting early on in the child's life, wishing to fairly directly get off on the child by working themselves into a frenzy while yelling or hitting the child, or stroking the child or getting the child to stroke them.

In the latter case, erotomania may predominate. The psychotic feels certain that he is loved, often by an eminent person—who may in this case be the analyst—and that eminent person is the one who is believed to have initiated the contact and relationship, not the patient. The libido here is experienced by the psychotic as coming from the analyst (or some other figure) and targets the analysand (Maleval, 2000, p. 367).[4]

In this second case, the analyst risks becoming viewed as either a persecutor or as someone who loves but probably also wants to use and sexually exploit the psychotic. In such cases, psychotics may feel that they have to allow themselves to be seduced and used sexually in order to survive, that they either have to offer themselves up to be beaten or killed by the analyst, or else attack the analyst directly.

The first of these two possible positions (number 1 above) involves what Lacan calls the *imaginary* dimension of human experience: idealization which is often quite instantaneous and based on very little information. It does not involve the attempt to discern what it is that allowed the person who is idealized to become a powerful and prestigious person in the world and then try to consider what qualities I myself have that could allow me to come to occupy a similarly powerful and prestigious position in the world, but rather simple imitation. In psychoanalytic jargon, we could say that it does not involve a symbolic identification, but rather a massive imaginary identification.

The second of these two possible positions (number 2 above) involves what is experienced by the psychotic as very *real* persecution and/or exploitation, real in the sense that it directly targets the psychotic's body.

Neither of these positions, then, leaves room for a *symbolic* transference, one based on the belief that the analyst knows something about what makes the patient tick. When neurotics situate the analyst as a subject-supposed-to-know—as someone who knows the why and wherefore of their problems, conflicts, and symptoms in life, who knows something that is of crucial interest to the patient—the kind of knowledge involved in the transference that grows out of this is thought to be formulable in words, and initially grows out of what the patient believes to be either in-depth study of human psychology or long experience of working with others on the analyst's part.

Many analysts noted early on that most psychotics do not seem to be terribly interested in the why and wherefore of their problems and conflicts. Rather than seeking some sort of abstract or articulable knowledge that helps them reconstruct their own history—in other words, how and why they got to be where they ended up, all the twists and turns of fate that led them into the predicaments they find themselves in today—psychotics can be understood to be seeking *a different kind of knowledge*. They may come to attribute that different kind of knowledge to the psychoanalyst, assuming he or she takes up the proper role ascribed to him or her in the analysis: someone who knows *how to do* certain things, knows how to get along in the world, for example, how to handle certain human passions, how to make a name for himself, how to negotiate social situations, school, work, friendship, sex, marriage, and so on. We will examine the exact nature of this *know-how* (knowing how to handle jouissance in all its varied forms: anxiety, panic, manic working, uncontrollable energy) further on.

Lacan, like most other psychoanalysts who have devoted quite a bit of time to working with psychotics, concluded that classical psychoanalytic interpretation aiming at interpreting the past or meaning-making either has no effect with psychotics or is considered intrusive, confusing, infuriating, or crazymaking by them and leads them to either break off the treatment or to take some kind of desperate action, such as self-harm, suicide, or even attacking the analyst. This is very different from the neurotic's "acting out," in which something the patient feels incapable of saying in the analysis, or feels the analyst does not want to hear, gets said through action. The French refer to what the psychotic does as a *passage à l'acte*, a desperate act; it is *not* an expression of the unconscious but a sign that the patient is falling apart, that the treatment is making him worse, not better.

Tempering jouissance

Whereas Lacan generally used the term "subject of the signifier" (*sujet du signifiant*) or "subject of the unconscious" (*sujet de l'inconscient*) in talking about neurotics—which we might also render as the "linguistic subject" and the "unconscious subject" respectively (or even "the signifier as subject" and "the unconscious as subject")—he began using a different term, especially for psychotics, in the late 1960s: *sujet de la jouissance*—"the subject of jouissance" or the enjoying or libidinal subject.⁵ One can provisionally equate jouissance and libido, considering how Lacan once defined jouissance in Seminar XVI: "jouissance [is] defined as everything related to the distribution of pleasure in the body."

The shift that occurred in Lacanian circles after his death was a reorientation of work with psychotics around helping them rein in their uncontained, unbounded energy, their sexual and aggressive thoughts that they feel are out of control and incomprehensibly all over the place. This reorientation involved the attempt to help temper, moderate, or tamp down the psychotic's unregulated jouissance.⁶ Whereas analysts seek to *interpret* the neurotic's libido, interpret what brings him jouissance and why, they seek to *temper* the psychotic's libido (Maleval, 2019, p. 11).

Indeed, Michel Sylvestre came, in 1983, to formulate the analyst's sole duty with psychotics as that of "managing the jouissance of which [his patient] makes [him] the keeper [*gardien*]" (1987, p. 138). The analyst must allow psychotics to *deposit* that jouissance at his doorstep, as it were, let them talk about it *ad nauseum*, and leave that talk—and even writings about it—behind in the analyst's consulting room at the end of the session. When manic energy and agitation come on outside of the session, the psychotic can—assuming the analyst allows this to occur—deposit it with the analyst, transfer it to him, send it to him in the form of writing, by jotting down, emailing, or even texting (for example) the words that the voices say to him (Darian Leader has patients text such things to him; personal communication).

As Michel Sylvestre put it, "the psychotic offers up his jouissance to the analyst so that the analyst will [set limits to it and] establish rules for it" (1987, p. 130). Psychotics are not grappling with a symbolic Other that judges them, has high expectations for their intelligence or other abilities, weighs them in the balance, and generally finds them wanting like neurotics are. This symbolic Other may well weigh neurotics down, torture them in many ways, make them feel worthless, and give them the impression that their accomplishments are paltry and their moral compass deficient. Psychotics are not grappling with a symbolic Other like that; rather they are grappling with a real Other that wishes to invade, consume, and/or destroy them. They may express some of the same concerns as neurotics that I just listed, but the battle at stake with the kind of Other they are engaged with involves all-out war, the nuclear option not being excluded. (It might be clearer not to capitalize the other with whom the psychotic grapples, but Lacan capitalizes it, for better or for worse, instead of restricting the use of Other with a capital O to the symbolic register. We might try to understand the capital O in psychosis as related to the sheer massiveness of this figure in the psychotic's life.)

Psychotics view the jouissance they experience as coming from this exploitative real Other who seeks to get off on or abuse him, and the analyst may well be repeatedly thrust into this role, even when he does everything he can to avoid that. As Michel Sylvestre put it, there's only one possible response to this: "block it" (*s'y opposer*; 1987, p. 132). We direct the treatment by countering or blocking the Other's jouissance, jouissance that the psychotic perceives to be coming from the Other, which here may be the analyst as well. We have to stop the patient from offering himself up as an object to be exploited or sacrificed by others. We have to do our best to dispel all of the psychotic's statements to the effect that we are trying to seduce or otherwise use him, doing our best to explain in very direct, clear language that this is not the case and that our goals and wishes are quite different from those he or she is imagining. We have to refuse all offers made by psychotics to serve us or sacrifice themselves to us. We have to do our best to distinguish ourselves in their minds from the real, exploitative Other whom they expect to enjoy at their expense. We have to strive to show as few signs as possible of any such enjoyment during sessions: neither titillation nor fury.

We also have to attempt to counter certain of their beliefs regarding other people in their entourage who they begin to believe are seeking to seduce or exploit them. We have to gently question the basis of their assertions and delicately try to suggest alternative readings of those people's behavior and comments, assuming, that is, that we truly believe they are misreading the intentions of those around them.

Whereas neurotics complain that they don't know what turns them on, that they don't like what turns them on, or that there are too many limits and restraints to their jouissance, psychotics complain of too much energy, excessive agitation, and overly intense sexual impulses and thoughts. This implies radically different approaches to treatment: the neurotic is asking for the knots in his desire to be untied, for certain inhibitions to be lifted, for certain superego prohibitions to be loosened so that he can finally enjoy himself a little bit, instead of finding satisfaction only in fantasy or in the distasteful form of his neurotic symptoms.

The psychotic is asking for inhibitions to be installed and for prohibitions to be reinforced, so that he can begin to calm down and live like other people seem to live.

In one case we work to assist the patient in attaining more jouissance, less tortured jouissance as it were, and in the other case we attempt to assist the patient in tempering his jouissance. These are very different projects indeed!

Providing structure

We have to agree to be situated as a prop or support for the search for words, for signifiers that can help organize the chaos in the psychotic's experiences (Maleval, 2000, p. 372). This is not a search for knowledge about the truth of the patient's history, for the patient himself believes that he has certainty about that—he is not opaque to himself, there is nothing unconscious in him, and his certainty about himself comes from his delusion and/or from the voices he hears—but a search for explanations for what seems inexplicable to him, for the thoughts and sensations that are experienced by him as "crazy."

It has often been noted that psychotics' lives have little to no structure, that they stay up all night, forget to eat or eat constantly, work for seventy-two hours straight or never get out of bed, and the like. And it has also been noted that many of them find solace in following strict orders and rules, the kind they are given in hospitals, monasteries, convents, the military, certain kinds of sports teams, and so on. Those rules and regulations help them regulate their own jouissance, help them structure their days and energy. (We might hypothesize that the ideals of the group or community help mask the missing Name-of-the-Father.) Such groups and institutions go much further in structuring their lives than can arise simply by coming to see the analyst several times a week in the same place and at the same time. But as many practitioners have pointed out, the time spent with us is often the only social contact psychotics have, and the session times we give them are the only things that structure their days.

Some of them have a tendency to live outside of time, not to know what day it is, or even what month or year it is. This is especially notable to us when we try to get a handle on their history, for many of them are unable to tell us when such and such an event occurred, whereas neurotics are often very good at or at least very concerned with telling us that such and such occurred when they were in second grade, and this other event occurred when they were in fourth grade, and so on. Neurotics' experience is anchored and recorded in generally recognized, shared symbolic time. Psychotics' experience is often far more adrift, and not tied to the culturally widespread ways of keeping track of time, whether in ages (France), grades (USA), seasons (agrarian societies), or what have you. Part of our work involves helping them establish external structures in which to situate themselves, structures in which they have contact with other people—that is, social bonds.[7]

How to work with delusions

By 1916, Freud had concluded that we cannot try to use what generally passes for reason or logic when faced with a patient's delusion, but that we must rather work from within the delusion. He came to realize that a delusion is an attempt at self-reparation, not something to be actively suppressed or destroyed. As he put it, "the paranoiac rebuilds [the beautiful world], not more splendidly, it is true, but at least so that he can once more live in it. He rebuilds it by the work of his delusions. *The delusional formation, which we take to be a pathological product, is in reality an attempt at recovery, a process of reconstruction*" (SE XII, pp. 70–71). To Freud's mind, a delusion was not what is often referred to today as a "thought disorder" but rather an attempt at cure.

Colette Soler refers to delusions as "a process of putting things into words [*significantisation*] ... by which the subject manages to develop and fix in place a form of jouissance that is acceptable to him" (1990, p. 28). In other words, a delusion weaves a story around this jouissance that renders it somehow palatable to him, there being an explanation for why he's experiencing it and why he is experiencing it in the form in which he is experiencing it. To grapple with that jouissance without any such story is highly destabilizing, for it seems to be coming out of nowhere, invading him from the outside for no apparent reason.

Psychotropic medications can be somewhat effective in tamping down that jouissance, moderating it, but they obviously do not in any way help weave a story about its why and wherefore. As Jean-Claude Maleval—whose work I am relying on extensively here without always citing his three fine books on psychosis (2000, 2011, 2019)—puts it, prior to the formulation of a delusion, the psychotic is "tormented by jouissance that is devoid of law or frame" (2011, p. 63).

Many psychoanalysts have concluded that the attempt to talk the patient out of his delusion is doomed to failure. Instead, we must listen to the account of it in all its details, without either confirming or denying its validity, and once the patient has acquired confidence in the analyst's willingness to listen to anything and everything without contradicting him, the analyst may be able to inquire about some of the evidence upon which the delusion was apparently built. This does not mean that the analyst directly calls it into question, but rather leans a bit on certain facets of it.

Now this is recommended only in cases in which the delusion has *not* reached the final stage of stabilization wherein the psychotic has delusionally recreated the world in such a way that he has an incredibly important role in it and considers himself to be the person who, unbeknownst to most others, is keeping the universe running—a world wherein he is God, God's wife, Napoleon, or the *éminence grise* of the CIA. It might be argued that at such a point, the curative process brought on by delusion formation has achieved its highest point of organization, its point of greatest stability.

The structure of psychotic difficulties

In addition to concluding that delusions are part of the self-curative process, Freud also concluded that it was generally not possible to interpret the psychotic's apparent psychical conflicts. Psychical conflict in Freud's theory of psychological functioning is the conflict between conscious and unconscious which, in neurosis, leads to symptoms that are "compromise formations," as he called them, compromises between unconscious wishes and conscious ideals, or between the id and the superego. But neurotically structured symptoms are not found in psychosis; indeed, a different definition of psychotic symptoms (such as the so-called elementary phenomena) is required, as well as a new way of thinking about their dynamics.

Lacan proposed that there is an unconscious in psychosis but that it does not function. As he put it in his study of James Joyce's work, Joyce "cancelled his subscription to the unconscious" (*désabonné à l'inconscient*).[8]

I, myself, would go a step further and say that there simply is no dynamic unconscious in psychosis and that the structure of the psychotic's difficulties is thus radically different from the structure of the neurotic's difficulties. The neurotic's problems involve a conflict between conscious and unconscious. Making the unconscious conscious *can*, in the case of neurosis, lead to curative effects. But the psychotic's problems do not involve a conflict between conscious and unconscious, and therefore the attempt to make the unconscious conscious is doomed to failure. What the analyst ends up doing is bringing to the psychotic's attention what the analyst himself believes *must be* unconscious in the psychotic, but which in fact is not. This, as a great many clinicians have pointed out, can be highly destabilizing to the patient. The attempt to interpret the unconscious in psychosis amounts to barking up the wrong tree—in a word, it is misguided.

Things to avoid doing

Freud's negative advice about working with psychotics

In addition to concluding that delusions are part of the self-curative process, and that it is generally not possible to interpret the psychotic's psychical conflicts, Freud also concluded that in treating psychotics, certain neurotic-looking defenses should not be disturbed as they may give way to or trigger a full-blown psychotic episode (Maleval, 2000, p. 389).

Ferenczi's negative advice about working with psychotics

Let us turn for a moment to Ferenczi. Ferenczi came to a number of conclusions about working with psychotics, based on his own clinical experiments with them:

1) Don't argue with the psychotic.
2) Treat delusions as possible rather than as absurd, especially at the outset.
3) Don't interpret dreams; let the psychotic do it himself.
4) Don't try to show the psychotic his "unconscious" for he believes nothing in himself is unconscious. Everything that would be unconscious in others, such as sexual and aggressive thoughts and impulses, are completely conscious in him (Lacan used a well-known French expression for this: *à ciel ouvert*, right out in the open, there for all the world to see; see *Écrits*, pp. 699 and 840 n. 825, 2).

Ferenczi recommended that we refrain from trying to show the psychotic "reality," refrain from insisting on "free association," and let the psychotic do his own interpreting. If we follow this advice, some positive attachment may ensue and we may avoid being situated as a persecutor (Maleval, 2000, pp. 390–391). Many analysts find their role with psychotics boring, as it requires even more self-effacement than work with neurotics does. Many therapists can barely stand the degree of self-effacement and abstinence generally required in work with neurotics, and truly cannot stand the still higher degree often required in work with psychotics.

Obsessive neurotics, for example, prefer it when the analyst plays dead, but the analyst must not agree to do so in their cases. The psychotic might prefer, in some sense, that the analyst not play dead, but then experiences him as enjoying too much, as enjoying at the patient's expense. In work with psychotics, the analyst must, if he is to *avoid* being associated with the real, exploitative Other, be perceived as enjoying as little as possible.

Lacan's negative advice about working with psychotics

Lacan himself did not provide positive recommendations about how to direct the treatment with psychotics. He confined himself to indicating a few things *not* to do. They are as follows:

1) *Don't have the psychotic lie on the couch*. This advice, provided by Lacan already in the 1950s, is often ignored even today, whereas it is quite clear that most psychotics prefer to have the visual prop of seeing the analyst in front of them. This allows them an image of a real person sitting across from them and thwarts their ability to imagine him as an ill-intentioned, ferocious creature as they might were he to be out of their direct line of sight. They may become suspicious of what the analyst is up to behind them on the couch, perhaps preparing to violate or kill them.

   To know who he is and experience himself as a whole person, the psychotic needs to see another person like himself in front of him. He can have a sense of himself while speaking only if his interlocutor is visibly and perhaps even physically present. "I see you over there as a whole person and we are talking and conversing like two whole people." There is a connection here with what Helene Deutsch called the "as if" personality: the psychotic can feel *as if* he is someone like the analyst and everyone else in such face-to-face interactions.

Whereas the neurotic may say the most profound things while not looking at the analyst, in the penumbra, or even in the dark, the psychotic may well become disoriented on the couch and fall apart, not knowing where his own voice is coming from. Insofar as the couch may be relaxing, it may allow unwanted thoughts and images to come to mind, whereas we are there to help him block out such unwanted thoughts and images. Psychotics have often found ways in everyday life to keep such thoughts and images at bay, but if they come to us for therapy and we tell them that we want them to allow any and every thought, image, and impulse to come to mind (i.e., free associate) and encourage them to do so by having them lie on the couch, they may find analysis to be an unbearable process. Some psychotics may do alright on the couch, but most do not. And when in doubt as to the patient's psychical structure early on in the treatment, it is best to continue face-to-face sessions for quite some time, meaning a year or more if necessary. (In general, analysts tend to rush patients to the couch before they are ready, but with potentially psychotic patients, they should especially take their time.)

It is, I think, worth emphasizing that *the couch does not an analysis make*. Analysis is defined by what you do with patients, not where they sit or lie in the office. I know plenty of analysts who have their patients lie on the couch but who are not working with them in a recognizably analytic way. Many of them might just as well be doing coaching or CBT.

2) We have to be careful about encouraging a psychotic to speak in a certain way in analysis, because analysis almost automatically thrusts the patient into the position of "I" in his discourse, which may be difficult for certain psychotics who feel they have no center, core, or foundation from which to speak. It is often easier for them to go along with what others say than to proffer and assume responsibility for ideas of their own. The very fact of taking a prepsychotic into analysis can occasionally trigger a full-blown psychosis.

The neurotic, on the other hand, may be pleased that he has finally encountered someone who asks him to speak in his own name, and who even perhaps repeatedly tells him, "So you've told me what other people around you want you to do—what about what *you* want to do? You've told me what other people around you think, but what do *you* think?" Certain neurotics may, for quite some time, couch many of the things they say in terms of "we"—referring to their family or coupled situation—or even "one" ("one feels that ..."), but we can safely encourage them to try to sift out what they believe and want from what those others believe and want. We must be careful about doing so with psychotics.[9]

3) Lacan's third recommendation was not to interpret using plays on words. Psychotics are averse to signifying ambiguity. In a recent session with one of my *neurotics*, the patient told me a dream in which she found a bunch of bugs or mollusks in her hair that she called "chitons." I didn't know what they were and asked her to explain and to tell me where she had heard about them, which didn't seem to take us very far in the interpretation of the dream until I said "cheat on." This struck her as highly significant and led to a long discussion of cheating on her part and on her partners' parts in all of her prior relationships.

Another patient who, at almost forty, is still extremely dependent on his parents, told me he had a dream in which there was a big storm that was leading to flooding, and he referred to the storm as a "monsoon." I encouraged him to associate to the word "monsoon" to no avail, and then attempted to break the word down for him as I pronounced it mon-soon, but he continued to come up emptyhanded. It was only when I said "you will become a man soon" that he burst out laughing.

A patient who recently gave up on a religion that had been extremely important to him for years reported a dream in which he "was being chased." It sufficed for me to ask him how he would spell chased/chaste for a long series of associations to ensue.

That is not the sort of thing Lacan would recommend we do in our work with psychotics. Many plays on words are simply not heard by them, whereas others may destabilize them. To their mind, what they say means one thing and one thing alone. There is no potential for something they say, or something that appears in a dream, to mean anything other than what it says at first sight, what it says right on the face of it. There is no slippage between signifier and signified, to put it in linguistic terms. Should the patient say something like, "that is where the lovers lie," fairly obviously referring to their physical position on a bed, nothing is gained by the analyst repeating the word "lie" to highlight the double meaning of the verb "to lie," as I did with a neurotic analysand. Should the analyst attempt to underscore it nevertheless, he may be met with incomprehension, stonewalling ("yes, yes, that's what I said"), and even anger if he persists.

Our assumption in our work with neurotics is that they inadvertently say more than they mean to say and we take it as our job to pick up on that extra meaning, which often goes in a completely different direction than the consciously intended meaning. With psychotics our assumption must be exactly the opposite: the psychotic says what she means and means what she says.

4) Don't make comments related to the absence or failure of the father in the psychotic's life history. Lacan's perspective is that no one in the child's life served what Lacan calls the "paternal function," "father function," or castrating function. No one laid down the law for the child, no one obliged the child to give up something in order to enter into the social world as most of us do by giving up our mothers as our primary libidinal object, it being made clear to us that she belongs to dad, not us, that she is *his* libidinal object. To highlight the absence of the father or the failings of the father figure in his life is to lead the patient toward a gaping hole in his universe and may trigger a psychotic episode.

5) Don't try to suggest that male psychotics are latent homosexuals. Freud believed that this was the case of Judge Schreber, for example, and true of male psychotics more generally. To try to suggest that they are latent homosexuals can have catastrophic results. This stems at least in part from the fact that trying to tell them anything about themselves of which they are unaware can be taken as a sort of violation. They believe they know themselves inside and out. They do not have the usual neurotic sense that there is something in themselves that is opaque to them, that there is some mystery hidden inside of them which they hope the analyst will help them uncover. Any attempt on the analyst's part to gesture toward or point toward something that is hidden or unbeknown to psychotics can be highly destabilizing.

The issue is still more complicated, however. Lacan formulated what he refers to as a "budding into woman" (*pousse à la femme*) that occurs in male psychotics (see, for example, *Autres Écrits*, p. 466), whereby their unbounded jouissance seems to lead them in the direction of the kind of jouissance they believe women have, and their delusions may lead them in the direction of seeing themselves as the perfect female partner for an eminent male figure, whether God, as in the case of Judge Schreber, the president of the United States, aliens, or what have you.[10]

If we take seriously Lacan's negative recommendations, we will see that whatever positive rapport we are able to establish with the psychotic will be very quickly eroded by having the psychotic lie on the couch, by encouraging or insisting on "free association," by highlighting double entendres or ambiguities in the patient's speech, by encouraging discussion of the patient's inadequate father, or by suggesting that the patient is a latent homosexual. The patient will come to feel that we are deliberately trying to destabilize or destroy him.

6) Lacan himself did not provide this further negative recommendation, but his followers did: knowing how difficult intimate encounters can be for psychotics, we should neither encourage nor discourage relationships that they form or are considering forming. Should we encourage them, they may feel that we are somehow trying to exploit them sexually, whether vicariously or otherwise (Maleval, 2000, p. 433).

The four stages of the development of psychosis

Jean-Claude Maleval, a Lacanian analyst who worked extensively with Lacan and who has devoted much of his career to studying the classics in psychiatry regarding psychosis and numerous contemporary case studies as well, has provided a sketch of the various stages in the development of psychosis that have been discerned over the last 200 years. If this were a purely academic exercise, I would not present it here, but since it can provide us guidance as to what we can do with patients we see who may be at one stage or another in the development of (full-blown, not pre- or ordinary) psychosis, I believe it is worth mentioning.

The stages Maleval (2011, pp. 115–116) outlines summarize and synthesize those provided by many of the classic writers in psychiatry such as Kraepelin, de Clérambault, and so on:

1) One, the "incubation period," is a stage in which we find perplexity, worry, and/or angst on the subject's part, often accompanied by uncontrolled energy and hypochondria. The subject has the impression that *something is wrong*, that something has changed, but he's not sure what it is. In this stage the subject may remain quite silent, preoccupied, pensive, and indeed incommunicable (catatonic or hebephrenic stupor).[11] The subject is faced with some kind of disruption,

disorganization, or "delocalization" of his jouissance which comes on more or less suddenly and he finds himself incapable of grasping why.

2) In the second stage, all of the patient's linguistic resources are mobilized (or mustered) to come up with an explanation for what is going on. He becomes certain here that he is targeted by a signification whose meaning is enigmatic to him—something Lacan calls a "signification of signification" in the *Écrits*, implying that he knows that there is a message that is specifically directed to him, but he doesn't know what it means. At this stage we often find intrusive thoughts, images, feelings, impulses, and unexplained sensations, bodily suffering, and hypochondria.

The intrusive thoughts generally take the form of what de Clérambault called "mental automatism" or "automatic thinking" in which the patient passively hears language speaking in his own head, all by itself, as it were, whether it simply echoes his own thoughts, or swears, curses, and says things the subject considers to be insulting and/or disgusting. It usually perplexes but also torments and ridicules the subject. Mental automatism is often accompanied by indistinct noises, whispering, the enunciation of the subject's actions ("she's doing this now") and thoughts ("he's thinking about this now"), explosive words, the mixing together of words, nonsense syllables, the silent replaying or recounting of memories in one's head, and a kind of involuntary commentary on actions and memories, questions and thoughts responding to each other. (Maleval considers such automatic thinking to be a sure sign [*signature*] of psychosis: we need no further corroborating signs to make the diagnosis.) Mental automatism is often accompanied by hallucinations, feelings of being possessed, jealousy, fighting with others, and contradictory explanations of things that happen.

The initial explanation of what is wrong that is usually alighted upon is that someone is trying to exploit or persecute the patient. In men, that someone is often a powerful father figure or a man with prestige and fame. Lacan noted, already in his Ph.D. dissertation in psychiatry, that persecutors are very often of the same sex as the patient, and in women the persecutor may be a prominent female singer, writer, actress, professor, politician, scientist, or CEO.

We might hypothesize that a word or a name is put here on the cause of the psychotic's troubles: a specific person is deemed responsible for what he is undergoing, or "the FBI" is plotting against him,

At this second stage, some sort of organization takes place, whereby there is no longer just a pure enigma but a construction, even if it remains somewhat mystifying. Lacan referred to this as the "fertile [or: productive or prolific, *féconde*] phase of the delusion" (2001, p. 63).

In cases of schizophrenia, on the other hand, no question is formulated, no specific enigma ever appears on the horizon, and no organization occurs. The schizophrenic senses that something is wrong or missing, that he has no foundation, no basis or yardstick for his being, but doesn't know what it is that he is missing.[12] Schizophrenics are the psychotics who are most likely to be thought of as having disorganized thinking or a "thought disorder," characterized by "loosened associations," non sequiturs, or even word or sound salad. (Our role with them could perhaps be to try to encourage the formulation of a question or specific enigma.)

In cases of melancholia, the psychotic experiences a disturbance in her world, but it does not appear to her to be coming from the Other. The melancholic feels that what is wrong in the world stems from something she *did*. She can locate no persecutor on whom to cast blame. The blame is cast upon herself, but she doesn't think there is something deep within herself that is wrong, something internal that needs to be fixed, but rather that she has *done* something that cannot be undone. Although sure it is her fault, she may not even be able to say what it is that she did.[13]

3) In the third stage (not reached by schizophrenics or melancholics), the persecutor is progressively viewed as an obscene figure who is destroying the world, whose jouissance is destructive, who is usurping the subject's rightful role in life. The subject may conclude at this point that it is the subject's responsibility to attack or even kill him or her.

The patient Lacan (1980) wrote about extensively in his doctoral dissertation, whom he called Aimée, went so far as to try to attack a famous actress with a knife, believing that woman was responsible for Aimée's problems but also setting a terrible example as a dissolute female in the France of the 1930s.[14]

We see in this third stage a kind of systematization of the delusional explanation of the subject's problem, which goes beyond simple persecution of the subject and concerns a disturbance being experienced by the entire country. The subject may find some solace already at this stage, because the obscene figure is thought to be ruining not just her life but the entire world.

4) In the fourth stage, and this is a stage that is reached by few psychotics—especially in our times owing to the extensive administration of psychotropic medications that affect the intellectual faculties—the subject makes his peace with the designs of this obscene figure, and appears to be flattered to have been singled out as his plaything or object of satisfaction. This is where we note the appearance of megalomania. Kraepelin called this "full-blown paraphrenia" or "systematic paraphrenia," and considered it to be the highest form of psychotic organization. At this point the subject may be content to be aware of his special position in the world as the targeted object of this incredibly powerful figure and feel no need to try to convince other people of it. He may be quite able to go on with his ordinary work and daily life, without letting the special position he believes he occupies interfere with such quotidian matters.

We might say that at this stage he has "consented to the Other's jouissance," has made his peace with the way in which this obscene figure wishes to seduce and/or exploit the subject. Indeed, the figure is no longer seen as obscene at this point, and is no longer felt to be persecuting the subject. In the case of Schreber, the subject concludes at this point that God requires of him a "constant state of jouissance" (Maleval, 2000, p. 422), constant voluptuous sensations, as he puts it, and he accepts that this is his fate as the wife of God. It was at this exact point that he was successfully able to argue for his release from the asylum he had been sent to and return home to his wife. I'm not trying to suggest that such consent to the Other's jouissance is necessarily a permanent solution, for we know that Schreber relapsed a number of years later and had to return to the hospital. But there were, I believe, about eight years of virtually total stabilization in his case.

Becoming the wife or elective plaything of such a figure is not the only solution characteristic of this stage: one may also become his servant, in some sense, spreading what one believes his message to be far and wide. Other solutions, too, are possible.

In the course of this four-stage process, we see the production of what Lacan calls a "delusional metaphor"—a delusional explanation of the subject's place in the universe. A delusion ties together words and meaning, giving sense to the world. This takes the place of what Lacan calls the "paternal metaphor," a metaphor or explanation that tells a child who he is and what his place is in a specific family, in a specific town, in a specific culture, religion, etc. Lacan postulates that this is precisely what is missing in psychosis: the paternal metaphor has not been instated in the subject's life and the subject is adrift, as it were, having no solid explanation for his being in the world. He has no anchor, no permanent compass in life. Psychotics often tell us that they feel they have no foundation, no base, no center, no ground on which to stand, no root in being, no place from which to speak or enunciate something in their own name.

For most of us, our place in a family and a community is at least to some degree established quite early on in life and is unshakable, apart from certain moments, especially in adolescence, where many of us wonder why we are here and what we are meant to do on this planet. We generally refer to this as an *"existential crisis."* At that time in life we are often looking for absolutes, absolute truth, absolute knowledge, absolute explanations, for the absolute origins of everything, whether that be the origins of human language or the origins of the cosmos. The adolescent's questions at that time often seem to be, "Why am I here?" "Where do I fit in?" "Am I of any significance in the world, in the larger scheme of things, or just a mote of insignificant dust?"

The budding psychotic is faced, by contrast, with what we might call an *"ontological crisis,"* and does not even know where the limits of his own body and being are. His quest for absolute truth is accompanied by weird sensations, aches and pains, intrusive sexual thoughts and impulses, and uncontrollable thinking. (None of this is characteristic of the adolescent's existential crisis.) The psychotic's thinking seems to go on all by itself, the subject just sitting back and watching. Not only does he fail to be situated in a social/cultural context—in other words in a symbolic frame—but his very body is undefined in certain ways, unbounded, uncastrated, uninscribed in the symbolic order. Lacan's notion here is that the delusional metaphor tries to do the same work for the psychotic as the paternal metaphor does for the neurotic.

What analysts can do at each stage

This four-stage schema should not be taken to imply that we want to encourage all psychotics to arrive at what Kraepelin called the highest form of psychotic organization by creating a full-blown delusional metaphor, for this involves recreating/reformulating the entire universe, making the whole cosmos over in the image of the delusion. Laying out these four different stages—which are not absolute but rather overlapping in practice—can give us some guidance as to the role we can usefully play at each point in time.

For example, at stage one (the "incubation period"), a combination of anti-anxiety medication and talk therapy may allow things to return to their earlier state. In many cases, that earlier state was more or less stable, and perhaps had been stable for decades, despite the absence of the paternal metaphor, despite the absence of the usual way of tying together the imaginary, the symbolic, and the real (i.e., the image of the body and its boundaries, language, and jouissance).[15] If the early stable state lasted thirty years, for example, talking and mild medication may be enough to keep the subject going more or less indefinitely, helping her absorb whatever minor bumps in the road arise along the way without too much trouble: conflicts with bosses, coworkers, partners, etc. It may be enough to persuade the psychotic to leave a job at which she is beginning to perceive her boss as a persecutor of some kind, or to dissuade the psychotic from entering into certain competitions, to calm things down and smooth things over. Of course, this approach may work once or twice, but not necessarily forever in cases in which the psychotic process has gone to a point of no return.

Another recommendation regarding technique can be seen to stem from this four-stage schematization: When we take someone we believe to be neurotic into analysis, but she very quickly begins to toy with the idea of having a different genealogy, we do not necessarily want to encourage this (Freud called it a new "family romance"; see Maleval, 2011, p. 132). For example, we need not encourage a woman who begins to think she is not the daughter of the people who raised her but rather the illegitimate daughter of the Grand Duke of Luxembourg, a direct descendant of the Kings of France, the Tzars of Russia, or of Napoleon to continue to elaborate on this particular line of thinking. We may want to steer the discussion away from it without directly contradicting it. Having entertained it for some time in the therapy, showing our willingness to explore it with her, we may be able to inquire about the evidence for each detail of it without professing not to believe her.

The idea here is that she may be at the very beginning of the process of constructing a delusional metaphor that will almost certainly take years to develop and involve a massive restructuring of her world. It may be more prudent in such a case to help her dissipate the enigma or question she is grappling with in a simpler and less taxing way for both her and her analyst.

Some MDs and psychiatrists do this quite inadvertently by providing psychotics—whom they generally do not recognize as such—with a diagnosis like ADHD, borderline personality disorder, or bipolar (and there are plenty of other ones available today, like fibromyalgia), thereby putting a name on the enigma. The diagnosis plugs up the gaping hole in meaning that has opened up for them, the patient receiving an explanation for something strange going on in his body or world from someone recognized to be an authority figure. That hole, where a question has arisen, has no words attached to it in the subject's own signifying system. Thought seems to break down there or be stymied, but it can be plugged up by a signifier that is provided by someone else.[16]

Early in my career I recall being incredibly frustrated in my work with a young man who was thoroughly convinced that the ADD diagnosis he had received from a psychiatrist explained all of his troubles in life. What I did not recognize at the time was that that label was probably doing a certain kind of work for him, serving as an explanation for what was going on for him. It was something I should have rolled with as opposed to questioning—not too incisively, but more than was undoubtedly called for—and having been so frustrated by it. I had failed to recognize that his was a case of what we might call untriggered psychosis, prepsychosis, or what is now often referred to in Lacanian circles as "ordinary psychosis"—in contrast to full-blown, extraordinary, florid psychosis, complete with auditory and visual hallucinations, delusions, etc. The psychiatrist he had consulted had, unbeknownst to himself, provided the patient with something that helped the patient keep body and soul together, perhaps even permanently. It's not every day that we psychoanalysts are able to do as much!

A number of psychotics believe that a certain form of bodily transformation will help restore order to their world, that there has always been something wrong with one of their limbs, and of course more commonly today, with their sexual organs. This may lead them to self-mutilate, or to request that a doctor remove an otherwise perfectly healthy limb—some doctors eventually agree to do so—or perform a sex-change operation. The belief here is that everything will fall back into place once their physical body has been transformed, and this often does indeed calm things down a great deal for certain subjects, at least for a while.

Regarding stage 4 (that of "systematic paraphrenia" or having consented to the Other's jouissance), many clinicians have noted that psychotics essentially feel no need or desire to talk to us at that point, feeling they have found their ultimate truth, found a way to keep body and soul together, word and meaning together (words don't seem to slip off of things as they did before), and have no need for us to help with that (Maleval, 2011, p. 132).

The transference that arises with those in stages 1 through 3 might thus be understood as simply positive regard, accompanied by the belief that talking with the analyst can help. This is not transference in the literal sense of a translation, transposition, or transferring something from the past onto the psychoanalyst, for often there was no one in the psychotic's history who attempted to help in any way. (Of course, such positive regard or good rapport is much more difficult to obtain and sustain with erotomaniacs.)

I mentioned earlier Malan's comment about transference: "the word has gradually become more loosely used for *any* feelings that the patient may have about the therapist." Now, as useless as this definition is to us in our work with neurotics—where we must distinguish between reactions to the analyst arising from projections as opposed to those arising from the way the analyst actually treats the patient—we might say that it fits our work with psychotics very nicely! When analysts do not situate themselves helpfully in their work with psychotics, but instead do things that their patients find to be destabilizing, they often hear remarks from their patients like, "You ruined my transference," or "You spoiled the transference." One of my supervisees spoke with me about a young patient she had been seeing for just a few months who informed her that he was getting worse and worse. Talking about his past and in particular about his father seemed to be making him fall apart, his paranoia that everyone was talking about him all the time getting more intense. The usual kind of work we do with neurotics can be quite destabilizing to such people.

What kind of Other we must incarnate in neurosis vs. psychosis

If we compare and contrast the kind of Other that the neurotic and psychotic are up against or dealing with, we find that the psychotic's Other is one who won't let go of him, wants to change him, make him over in his own image, and perhaps even absorb him (Maleval, 2000, p. 441). The neurotic's Other, by contrast, is usually a figure who did not, to the patient's mind, provide enough recognition and love, leaving him always wanting more and feeling that what he got was inadequate, that he was ripped off, that he got a bum deal in life. The neurotic is desperately looking for a sign that he is special or important to the analyst, trying to read every little gesture, breath, comment, willingness to accommodate schedule changes, and so on as signs of special consideration. The psychotic, by way of contrast, is convinced that he is a unique object of interest to the analyst because the analyst intends to exploit him, whether sexually or otherwise (Maleval, 2000, p. 424).

The neurotic can usually say, at least after a while in analysis, what he wants from the analyst: to get him to stop drinking, smoking, looking at porn, going to prostitutes, feeling so anxious, being so unsure of herself, so panicky in social settings, etc. The psychotic is more likely to say something like "I am hoping for something from you," but without being able to articulate what that is (Maleval, 2000, p. 443).

The psychotic is not grappling with a symbolic Other, and our only handhold or leverage point is the imaginary register. We must attempt to support whatever feasible-sounding initiatives psychotics make based on ideals they have or form that seem to us to be compatible with contemporary social life, whether those initiatives involve becoming members of the helping professions, learning a trade, engaging in artistic activities, writing, or what have you (Maleval, 2000, p. 431). Children and adolescents who idolize certain superheroes can be guided in their idealization of those figures away from their more violent proclivities and toward their espoused commitments to honor, justice, friendship, and the like (Peoc'h, 2022). In this way, we work with whatever pre-existing ideals the patient may have formed in the course of life, and whatever pre-existing ideal figures he may have come to admire, and attempt to separate the wheat from the chaff, as it were—that is, strip away the characteristics of those ideal figures that may get the psychotic into trouble and showcase and bolster the ones that may be helpful.

Here we see how different our approach should be with neurotics and psychotics. With neurotics we never presume we know anything about what might be for their own good, and allow them to sift that out and work that out for themselves. If we attempt to steer them based on our own worldviews, it may be appreciated by some at first, insofar as it relieves them of responsibility for their own lives, but will often later be resented and viewed as an attempt to interfere with their own autonomy, just like their parents and/or others did.

With psychotics, on the other hand, we have to use our own hopefully enlightened and flexible judgment about what may be useful and helpful to the specific patient at hand, trying to steer her away from things that are likely to lead her to self-destruct.

The analyst operates here as "the best friend you never had"—a friend who really cares about your own good, not about his/her conception of what is good for everyone. The analyst strives to act here in certain ways like the best friend you could ever possibly hope for: a friend who encourages your pursuits not for his own purposes or profit but, to the highest degree possible, in what he assesses to be your best interest. Such an assessment cannot be made quickly or once and for all; it requires extensive knowledge of the analysand and must be open to continual revision.

In our work with neurotics, we may well realize that they are harming themselves by certain of the activities they engage in, but the attempt to persuade them or steer them away from them is generally pointless. We have to bring them to the point where they themselves decide to change what they are doing. With psychotics, we have to use whatever leverage we are able to muster from the positive transference to oppose the psychotic's self-destructive activities, whether they involve drugs, suicidal gestures, self-harm, persistent thoughts of harming others that may grow out of watching violent TV shows and movies, or playing violent video games. All we can do in such cases is impress upon the patient that engaging in those activities is likely or even certain to jeopardize the continuation of the treatment (Maleval, 2000, p. 445).

This does not mean that we cannot affirm their pre-existing beliefs that certain behaviors and activities are bad or perverse and their attempts to struggle against or turn off obsessive sexual and aggressive ideas. We don't offer our own beliefs, but we can affirm theirs. We don't adopt the kind of permissive attitude which we generally adopt in our work with neurotics, hoping to help them free themselves from various inhibitions they have to doing things they want to do. We don't, for example, ask psychotics what is so bad about such and such or suggest that "all is permitted."

Nor do we tell them that certain activities are not good for them. Such comments have no effect since the patients are deriving a kind of unbridled jouissance from them, which they may experience as good, if not great, at least in certain respects. We do not appeal to abstract symbolic notions like what is good for you and what is bad for you, but rather what is likely if not sure to interrupt the treatment. (We sometimes have to do that with perverts as well.)[17]

Comments about this being good for them, and that bad, have been made to them all their lives by their parents, in any case, and to speak to them like everyone else does is simply to encourage a conflation of the analyst with parental figures who were experienced, generally speaking, to be persecutory or exploitative. In our work with psychotics, we need to do our best to avoid becoming associated in any way with parental figures in the psychotic's mind.

In neurosis such associations between parental figures and the analyst are inevitable, often being based on just one or two physical or symbolic features—having the same eyebrows, wearing the same kinds of clothes or glasses, using similar idiomatic expressions, for example. The association is rarely as global or massive as it becomes in psychosis, and the projection onto the analyst that he is like a parental figure can be fruitfully discussed in the analysis itself, usually leading to an attenuation of that association and a recognition that the analyst is not, in fact, just like one of the neurotic's parents.

The way the psychotic uses us is as a witness or reassuring advisor or counselor of some kind, one who does not get off, who is not titillated by salacious details in the patient's speech, not excited like his parents might have been. The psychotic wants someone to listen to his certainties without disapproving or contradicting them. We tolerate his certainty without being complicit or agreeing with the delusion, if one has already formed. We allow the psychotic to situate us as a mostly silent partner or accompanist in the work of elaborating a delusion. If we stupidly believe it is in his interest not to have a delusion and try to directly counter it, we may well become experienced as persecutors.

Ordinary psychosis: what it is and how to treat it

I will conclude this discussion with what has become known in Lacanian circles as "ordinary psychosis"—in contrast to extraordinary, florid psychosis, complete with auditory and visual hallucinations, delusions, and so on. In the past, ordinary psychosis went by numerous different names, including untriggered psychosis, prepsychosis, cold psychosis [*psychose froide*], and white psychosis [*psychose blanche*]. The idea here is that we encounter people who *have not had a psychotic break*, a break in which the more usual signs of full-blown psychosis are seen by one and all, but whose psychical structure is nevertheless psychotic.

Lacanians do not endorse the idea that someone can be psychotic at certain moments in time and neurotic at others, but rather that in order to have a psychotic break, one had to have had a specific psychical structure all along. What do I mean by "all along"? I mean starting, in any case, by the end of childhood, which seems to be the point after which psychical structure is more or less set in stone. As is language acquisition, not that surprisingly, it having been observed that children who were not introduced to language by eight to nine years of age fail to assimilate language thereafter.

It has often been found that those who have psychotic breaks in their twenties, thirties, forties, or even later, showed signs of language disturbances of various kinds and withdrawal from social contact going back to at least adolescence. As adolescents, their peculiarities were often chalked up in their social milieu to shyness, embarrassment, inability to concentrate, general intellectual slowness, and the like. Teachers and peers noted their oddness, rigidity of thought, or adoption of the beliefs of those around them, as well as their fascination with cryptograms, crossword puzzles, and other word games emphasizing the letters in words as opposed to their meanings. People also often noted their apparent lack of a sense of humor, failure to get jokes that involve plays on words, and so on. Initial hints of paranoia may have arisen after first smoking marijuana, but persisted even when not smoking. And family members and friends may have noticed that they looked at themselves in every reflecting surface, often for very long periods of time, studying their image in the mirror. This is known in psychiatry as "the sign of the mirror" (Maleval, 2011, p. 130) and is correlated with psychotic structure, often being an early outwardly visible sign of it.

The psychoanalytic explanation for the latter is that when one has no symbolic foundation for one's being, when one has not fully entered into the symbolic order, one of the only other ways to assure oneself that one exists and of one's characteristics is via the visual image of oneself seen in such reflective surfaces. The sign of the mirror may also appear in what I earlier called stage one of the development of psychosis, when the subject begins to feel that something is wrong, that something has changed, without knowing what. The subject then looks again and again in the mirror to see whether what has changed is visible in the mirror and can thus take on some sort of consistency. You may recall that Judge Schreber examined himself for hours in the mirror, looking for signs of his transformation into a woman. Extremely subtle signs of transformation may be "detected" by certain patients at this stage, signs that no one else can see. But the patient may also fail to recognize himself, not really knowing who he is, his vague sense of himself not matching the image he sees in the mirror.

We might say that the psychotic structure manifested by one or more of these characteristics remains subclinical, in the sense that no one seems to take much notice of them or consider them to be worrisome or to require treatment (Maleval, 2019, p. 34). And that structure may remain quite stable and never give rise to a break or breakdown of any kind. There are plenty of people who go through life for multiple decades with very rigid views, often very conformist views, and who are described by others as being more normal than anyone else, as the most normal person you could ever meet.

Psychoanalysts tend to be very frustrated with such patients when they consult us for stress, anxiety, sleeplessness, and so on, finding the lack of dialectic in their thinking infuriating. The attempt to interpret slips, dreams, and daydreams with them falls flat; they often provide few if any associations, and either do not comprehend or become agitated by or angry at interpretations provided by their analysts. They do not seem to be open to any sort of recognizably psychoanalytic work.

Some of them, on the other hand, may endorse any and every view the analyst expresses, ostensibly adopting all of the analyst's ideas as their own, but never provide any further confirmation or further interpretation of what has happened in the course of their lives. Psychologists tend to pejoratively refer to such patients as "compliant" or "overly compliant." In their cases, "improvement" may occur as long as the treatment continues, but the patient may quickly conform to someone else's beliefs and lifestyle once the treatment ends. Styles of dress, drug use, musical tastes, and politics may change as often as the patient changes towns, jobs, and friend groups, without the patient seeing any contradiction among them or feeling he needs to justify those changes.

In this latter case, we can postulate that the patient is able to hold himself together by assimilating the identity provided by a certain group—whether it is that of indie rock musicians, law enforcement, goths, the military, sects, or what have you. These are ready-made identities that they can slip into, as it were, and which may provide them a somewhat solid sense of self for a period of time. Trouble may arise when they feel obliged or forced to change groups, whether their stint in the military (tour of duty) ends owing to no initiative of their own, or something seems to go wrong in the group they had been a part of. But some of them can be chameleon-like and fairly easily move from one group identity to another. They use the image of another person or a group of people as a prop for their own sense of themselves (something seen in the earliest constitution of the ego prior to the full-blown mirror stage; see Fink, 2016, chapter 5). Those who don and doff identities like hats are often considered to be impostors.

Others develop extremely strong identifications with just one person or character, whether a cartoon character, a character in a film or book, or even an avatar in a video game. Analysts may be frustrated that such patients do not seem to be "their own person," but constantly refer everything back to the person or character with whom they identify. This is known in some Lacanian circles as "overidentification," and it can serve as a way of solidifying the patient's ego in cases where no internal solidification has occurred, the kind that occurs owing to the assimilation of the unary trait during the mirror stage. They act in the world "as if" they were that character. Helene Deutsch called such people "schizoid," and claimed that schizophrenia sometimes ensues.

Attempts by the analyst to disrupt that identification or directly challenge it can be highly destabilizing to the patient, and analysts would do well to strive instead to work with it, emphasizing whatever positive, constructive qualities that character may possess and downplaying the more negative, destructive qualities.

Such overidentification can occur with social roles as well, subjects becoming the perfect employee, the perfect soldier, the perfect mother, etc. Such identifications can hold up extremely well for considerable periods of time, as long as contradictory demands are not made of them by their superiors and they are not worked to death by their superiors. In the case of a woman who overidentifies with her role as a mother, trouble may ensue when her children grow up and leave home, one possible solution for her being to adopt other children or take in foster children.

The analyst in such cases engages in a conversation with the patient as a fellow human being [*semblable*] who is willing to make use of whatever the psychotic already has developed by way of compensations in life, whether they involve an extremely strong identification with a certain group or person, an artistic practice, a lifestyle, a style of dress, or the adoption of a new name and possibly even a new sex, which will, they feel, somehow make everything right. The analyst here is anything but conventional and conservative in what she believes can work for the patient in the world around us. The analyst must help him insert or reinsert himself into society, being willing to go with whatever the patient brings.

The conclusive diagnosis of ordinary psychosis requires an accumulation of converging clinical signs. There is probably no one sign that in and of itself can provide us with certainty as to the diagnosis (apart, perhaps, from the sign of the mirror).

We find ordinary psychotics among hoarders, cutters, and fire setters. Hoarders have rather unusual relationships to their own bodies, preferring to spend nothing on heat or food, in other words on necessities, all of their attention being devoted to the objects they stock up and keep forever. Cutters who self-mutilate may be attempting to somehow provide limits to their own bodies, or make themselves feel that they inhabit their own bodies. They may feel at some distance from what they are doing while cutting, at one remove from themselves, and attempt to somehow bridge that distance. Some feel no pain, as if their bodies were dead. Others work or run until they experience pain because that pain in some way makes them feel they are in their bodies. Fire setters often have no idea why they did what they did and when asked say, "I don't know, something came over me."

Ordinary psychotics often have few friends, few attachments, and find it hard to work in groups. Their affect is often blunted, and some of them say they have never been in love, and in fact don't even know what love is. Those around them may express shock if and when they decompensate or burn a house down. "He seemed completely normal," they protest.

In conclusion

Not everyone needs to take psychotics into analysis. It requires a different way of working for which not everyone has the vocation. Someone who works only virtually may prefer not to take on psychotics; in many cases, however, the diagnosis is only confirmed after the analysis is well underway. The same is true of sadists and masochists: we mustn't refuse to study such structures and imagine how we can work with them, but no one individual is obliged to take them into analysis.[18]

MIS-READING

CHAPTER 3

The many faces of the imaginary

(This paper was presented as a keynote address, at the invitation of Dan Collins and Rolf Flor, at the APW conference "On the Imaginary" held in Boston October 11–13, 2013.)

The imaginary is discussed at many different periods in Lacan's work and goes by various names at different times: the mirror stage, the ego, resistance, dual or dyadic relations, semblance (above all in Seminar XVIII), meaning (*sens*, especially in Seminars XXI and up), intuition, and consistency. In contributing to our work on the imaginary here this weekend, I will discuss just a couple of Lacan's early formulations regarding the imaginary.

The overriding importance of images

Lacan's early work on the imaginary grew out of his study of ethology (that is, animal behavior), most notably that of the work on grasshoppers by R. Chauvin (1941) and on the sexual maturation of pigeons by L. Harrison Mathews (1939). Their research was discussed in Lacan's papers entitled "Some Reflections on the Ego" (1953) and "Remarks on Psychical Causality" (*Écrits*, pp. 189 and 190–191). Lacan was also quite familiar with Konrad Lorenz's earliest work on fish, geese, and other animals (see, for example, Lacan, 2013, p. 12).[1] These ethological studies emphasize the importance of images for triggering significant developmental processes. For example, in the migratory locust, a solitary individual changes into a gregarious one when it sees the characteristic shape and movements of another member of its own species. In a second example, a female pigeon matures sexually upon seeing (not simply hearing and/or smelling) another pigeon, or upon seeing just a rough cut-out facsimile of a pigeon, or even upon seeing its own reflection in a mirror. An example Lacan does not cite, as it had probably not yet been studied at the time, is that of the whydah, a kind of parasitical bird that lays its eggs in other bird species' nests, leaving the feeding and raising of its young to foster parents. The "female whydah becomes reproductively active and ovulates only when she sees the reproductive activity of members of her particular host species" (Avital & Jablonka, 2000, p. 129). The field of ethology has found many more such examples in the seventy years since Lacan first published his work on the formative nature of images in his paper on the mirror stage (*Écrits*).

The importance of images in the animal kingdom can be further illustrated by the fact that in many bird species,

> a female looks for a mate with the most extravagant traits—the most colorful male, the biggest, the strongest, the one presenting the most elaborate and demanding ritual. In some [polygamous] birds, including the peacock and a variety of game birds and waders, males gather together in advertising congregations called "leks," where they show off, and females come to look them over, compare them and choose the best male. When the female preference is not innate, and discernible markers of male quality change with circumstances, inexperienced young females may face a problem: they cannot easily tell who is the superior male. In such cases, young females seem to observe the behavior of older and more experienced females, and copy their choices. […] The consequence for males is that an already successful male becomes increasingly more popular! (Avital & Jablonka, 2000, pp. 143–144)

Further on, the same authors comment that,

> The peahen chooses the peacock with the largest and most colorful tail, and middle-aged males, who have proved their ability

to survive, are often preferred to young, inexperienced ones. The brightness of the male's plumage reflects his health, since parasite-infested males tend to have dull plumage. [...] The brightness of the plumage is also an index of fertility, because it is often correlated with high concentrations of [...] testosterone. [...] Attractiveness *per se* is also important. [...] A female who chooses a male considered to be attractive will probably have attractive sons. These sons will attract and mate with many females, and consequently produce many grandchildren. If attractiveness does not reduce the survival of the males too much, then in each generation the most attractive males, and the females most susceptible to their charms, will be selected. This can sometimes lead to evolutionary escalation—to exaggerated female preferences and inflated male traits that have more to do with fashion than with quality. The magnificent tail of the male peacock [which is sometimes so big and heavy that he can barely fly] and the complex and lengthy song of the nightingale are famous examples of traits that probably evolved both as extreme advertisements of genetic worth and as escalated fashions. It seems that both good sense and fashionable structures drive female preferences. (pp. 144–145)

After quoting such remarks, I perhaps hardly need to raise the question whether human beings are as affected by or dependent upon images as animals are, but I will anyway.

But first let me point out how much more complicated attraction is in human beings, the "right" or most desirable partner often having such symbolically determined characteristics as being from a part of the world or a religious background once spoken of in glowing—or alternatively—in deprecating terms by a parent; being about to leave the country, such that any relationship with that partner will almost certainly be short-lived or difficult; being already taken, indeed already in a committed relationship with one's best friend and thus off-limits, but oh-so-exciting; being the exact opposite of one's parents in political viewpoint; the possibilities are endless!

Returning to the question whether human beings are affected by or dependent upon images, Lacan certainly points to the crucial role of *self*-images in the formation of the human ego. But I suspect that he would be less sympathetic to the overwhelming importance granted to images by large numbers of psychologists, human sociobiologists (who now generally prefer to be known as evolutionary psychologists or evolutionary anthropologists), ethologists, and so on. A great many clinicians are enamored—not unlike much of the untrained general public—of the notion of *body language* and believe that it is not only possible but also crucial to know how to read it well. The ethologists lend them support here, Darwin perhaps first in line, by attempting to show that certain facial expressions and body postures have the same meaning in all members not only of *Homo sapiens* but in other mammalian species as well, his idea obviously being that humans inherited such expressions and postures from their animal ancestors.

Let me begin with a few basic examples: dominance and submission postures have been studied extensively by ethologists, owing to their importance in establishing hierarchies and pecking orders in animal groups and in the avoidance of constant conflict within such groups. Here is an example from a recent book on *Animal Social Complexity* (de Waal & Tyack, 2003, p. 278).

In the upper part of Figure 3.1, we see the zebra to the right demonstrating a submissive posture toward the zebra to the left. Note that

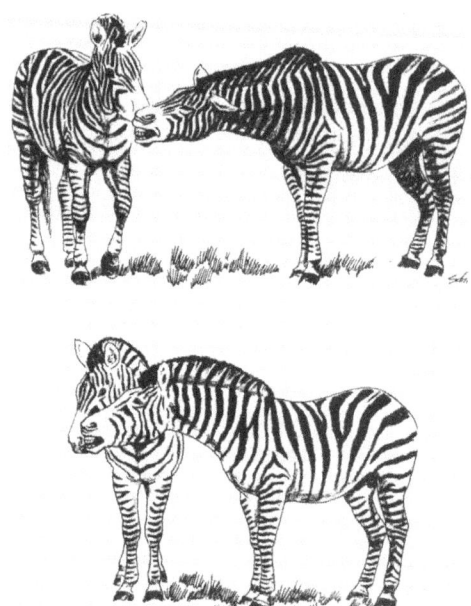

Figure 3.1: Zebras (upper section, contrasting with body posture in the lower section)

THE MANY FACES OF THE IMAGINARY   81

the neck is bowed compared to the more ordinary greeting posture shown in the lower part of the figure (we are led to presume that the greeting posture is one among friends, if not among equals), and it is but one short step for many ethologists and psychologists from the zebra's bowed neck to stooping postures and the bowing of heads in human beings.[2]

Note, too, in the upper part of Figure 3.1, that the zebra to the right seems to have a sort of pained smile on its face. It appears that a great deal of ink has been spilled in the field of animal behavior studies about the origin of so-called smiling in mammals, smiling having for many centuries apparently been considered (perhaps since Aristotle) to be an attenuated form of laughter, or a stage on the way to laughter (the latter being characteristic primarily of human beings: as Rabelais said, *le rire est le propre de l'homme*; but some have tried to find laughter in chimps too). Yet a number of ethologists have gone to rather great lengths to demonstrate that smiling with teeth bared derives phylogenetically from a fear response. It arises spontaneously, according to them, in many species as a demonstration to another member of the same species that one is afraid of that member and has no intention to attack that member.

In short, they argue that Darwin was wrong in thinking that the bared-teeth grin of a Sulawesi macaque was an expression of being pleased (see Figure 3.2). Darwin argued this in his study of the emotions entitled *The Expression of the Emotions in Man and Animals* (1872). Others claim that it is instead an expression of fear or a message to a

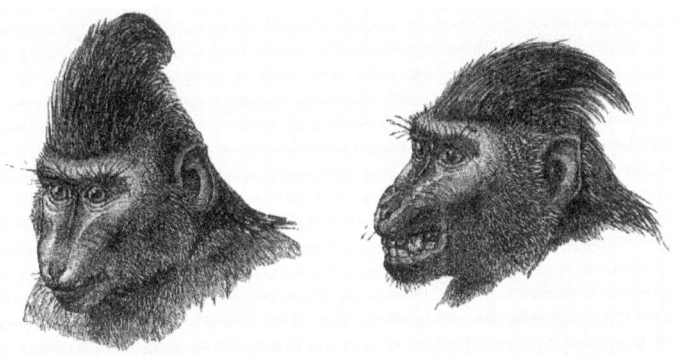

Figure 3.2: Sulawesi macaque

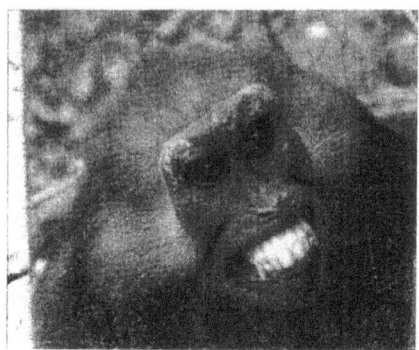

Figure 3.3: Bared teeth

potential aggressor that one accepts the other's dominant position and has no intention to attack or resist (see Figure 3.3).³

Whether smiles originated as fear responses or not, this kind of thinking follows directly from Darwin's in his book on the emotions. In one instance, Darwin showed photographs (provided by a certain Dr. Duchenne) of an old man's face to more than "twenty educated persons of various ages and both sexes, asking them, in each case, by what emotion or feeling the old man was supposed to be agitated" (Darwin, 1872, pp. 16–17). The results he reported as follows:

> Several of the expressions were instantly recognised by almost everyone, though described in not exactly the same terms; and these may, I think, be relied on as truthful [...]. On the other hand, the most widely different judgments were pronounced in regard to some of them. This exhibition was of use in another way, by convincing me how easily we may be misguided by our imagination. (p. 17)

Despite the only partial success of this particular experiment, Darwin went on to survey people the world over to test whether "the same movements of the features or body express the same emotions in several distinct races of man" in view of determining whether such expressions are "innate or instinctive" (p. 17) as opposed to cultural and thus learned. He initially entertained the hypothesis that "Conventional expressions or gestures, acquired by the individual during early life, would probably have differed in the different races, in the same manner as do their languages" (p. 17). In particular, he asked his correspondents whether astonishment, shame, indignation, contemplation, low spirits,

THE MANY FACES OF THE IMAGINARY   83

obstinacy, contempt, disgust, sulkiness, guilt, jealousy, and agreement were expressed in their parts of the world as he believed they were expressed in British culture at the time. Despite entertaining, in theory, the hypothesis that faces and gestures mean different things around the globe, his biologicist presumption was that more or less all of his contacts on different continents would describe the expression of such emotions, as experienced by the aborigines and other non-European peoples in their necks of the woods, in much the same way. He attempted to get his respondents to give specific detailed descriptions of the countenance corresponding to any particular emotion or frame of mind, and concluded that:

> It follows, from the information thus acquired, that the same state of mind is expressed throughout the world with remarkable uniformity; and this fact is in itself interesting as evidence of the close similarity in bodily structure and mental disposition of all the races of mankind. (p. 19)

This strikes me as a rather disingenuous conclusion, but psychologists like Paul Ekman (see Figure 3.4) have made a career out of arguing that a large number of human emotions are universally expressed in

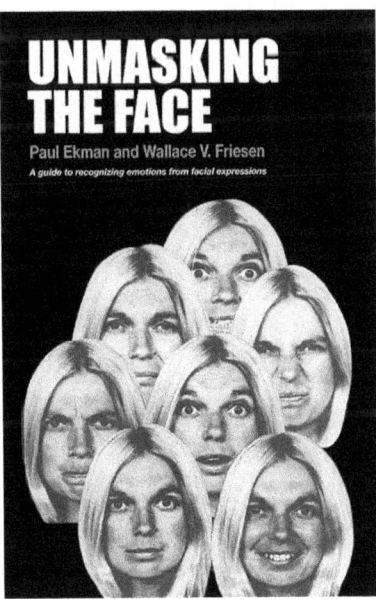

Figure 3.4: Cover of Ekman's book *Unmasking the Face*

84   MISS-ING

the same way by all people, regardless of socioeconomic class, cultural origin, religious background, and native tongue.

Given the myriad differing interpretations of virtually everything in our world on the part of different subjects, it would seem to me to be far more likely that different people would interpret pictures of people's faces in a wide variety of ways, depending on their backgrounds; and that one and the same person might interpret the same facial expression or bodily posture in different ways at different times depending on the particular moment at which they are asked to interpret it, given the degree to which projection is often at work in our interpretations of other people's states of mind, such interpretations constituting a kind of Rorschach test.

I would suspect that whereas it might be likely that in the animal kingdom, certain faces or expressions are rather instinctually based and thus have a somewhat well-defined meaning for the majority of the members of a particular species, in the human world it is far less likely. This has not stopped researchers in psychology from attempting to define for us the various faces and expressions that reflect well-known human emotions like anxiety, fear, horror, joy, sadness, etc. I cannot claim that I have read all of this literature, but, being as prone as anyone else to dwelling in the imaginary, I have looked at plenty of the pictures included in such studies purporting to show us the universal image of disgust, for example, and remain profoundly skeptical of their conclusions (see Figures 3.5, 3.6, and 3.7 and try to guess what emotion each supposedly portrays; for Ekman's answers, see footnote 4).[4]

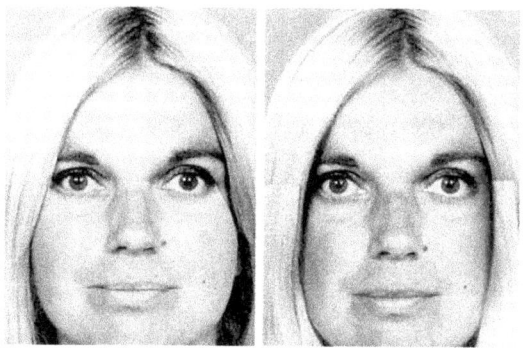

Figure 3.5: Guess the emotion

THE MANY FACES OF THE IMAGINARY   85

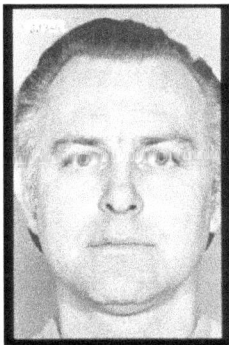

Figure 3.6: Guess the emotion

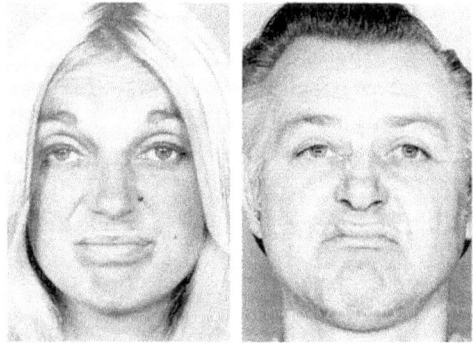

Figure 3.7: Guess the emotion

Luckily for us, there are researchers in other fields, like anthropology and even business, who have spent significant periods of time in foreign countries and have recognized the degree to which facial expressions and gestures mean rather different things in different countries. Here is a short list of books that indicate how different human gestures—whether hand, facial, or bodily—are in different cultures:

- *Italian Without Words,* by Don Cangelosi and Joseph Delli Carpini
- *The French Way: Aspects of Behavior, Attitudes, and Customs of the French,* by Ross Steele
- *Body Language in Business: Decoding the Signals,* by Adrian Furnham and Evgeniya Petrova
- *Cultural Intelligence: Living and Working Globally,* by David C. Thomas and Kerr Inkson

- *Understanding Cultural Differences: Germans, French and Americans*, by Edward T. Hall and Mildred Reed Hall
- *Culture Shock! Korea*, by Sonja Vegdahl Hur and Ben Seunghua Hur
- *Cultural Anthropology*, by Conrad Phillip Kottak
- *Gestures: The Do's and Taboos of Body Language Around the World*, by Roger E. Axtell.

Such works go a long way toward suggesting that postures and gestures form a true language tied to human language. Stated more accurately, there are many different gestural languages in different countries that are tied to the different languages spoken in those countries. As Lacan says in Seminar I, "a human gesture is more closely related to language than it is a manifestation of motor activity" (p. 255, trans. modified).

But let us suppose, for the sake of argument, that at least certain human emotions are expressed in some quasi-universal way. Why, we might ask, are psychologists so interested in demonstrating this? As Lacan put it in the early 1950s, their goal seems to be to find something surer to work from than patients' potentially lying speech. In other words, finding that they are unable to easily grasp what their patients say, or being uncertain whether or not to believe it, they seek something more "rock solid" upon which to base their understandings of their patients. Whereas speech can dissimulate and lie, they hope to find something that is not ambiguous or deceptive, something that would allow them to place psychotherapeutic work on a firm scientific basis. How do you know that your patient is depressed? It suffices to look at his face to know (see Figure 3.8), for his face corresponds to one

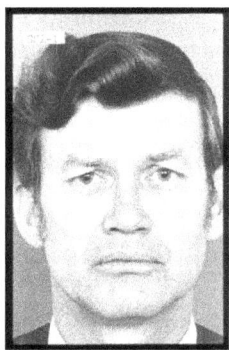

Figure 3.8: Sadness

of the six or seven universal emotions, one of which is, according to this theory, sadness.

Diagnosis then becomes a snap or at least a no-brainer: you take some pictures and compare the pictures with the ones found in the manuals—no problem. What you then do about the depression is another matter, but with the invention of antidepressants in more recent decades, at least one possible therapeutic course of action is "no-brainerly" indicated.

Language is, as Lacan indicated, a wall or barrier between us. It allows us to convey certain things but also to dissimulate, obfuscate, and throw off the scent. If we pay attention to the patient's speech alone, how are we ever to have an assured understanding of the patient? Lacan, as is well known, following in Freud's footsteps, provided us with many means by which to see through the patient's rhetorical strategies to glimpse something that the patient may be deliberately or not so deliberately keeping vague or out of sight. Speech, Lacan teaches us, may be confusing and obscure, never more than half-telling the truth, never revealing more than part of the truth, but facial expressions and body postures are no better, providing us with nothing like direct access to the patient's feelings, frames of mind, or mood states.

If they did give us direct access, how could we ever be deceived by people's facial expressions and body postures, which it seems we often are? Is it simply that we have not learned to read them properly, as Paul Ekman would argue? Or is it that those, too, can be simulated? An actor can, after all, put on a face or expression, or adopt a bodily stance, with which to make us believe he is feeling something he is not. And aren't we all sometime actors on the stage of life?

Note that among ethologists there is debate as to whether such faces or expressions are simply messages one sends to other members of one's species or whether such faces and expressions should be understood as genuinely reflecting the animal's emotions or inner states. In other words, we find in the ethological camp behaviorists for whom bodily postures and facial expressions are behaviors that need not be and perhaps even must not be interpreted as corresponding to some inner emotion or affect, and others who believe that such postures and expressions necessarily correspond to the animal's inner emotions. It is perhaps the behaviorists who could more easily accept the idea that an animal could potentially pretend to be submissive or fearful by engaging in the properly submissive body posture or giving the bared-teeth grin, only to attack as soon as the other party had relaxed and was no longer on guard!

This is obviously a strategy adopted by certain human beings—hide your game, don't show your cards, act the most politely to those you most hate, act the most coldly to those you most love, etc. But we do find a certain number of faking games in the animal kingdom—things that are done for show and to fake others out. Consider the following:

In certain bird species, there are helpers (birds of breeding age that do not currently have a mate) who help a specific couple feed their young, especially when mates are scarce. These helpers are more likely to mate subsequently with the young they themselves help to rear (Avital & Jablonka, 2000, pp. 217–222). However: "Juvenile birds help the breeding pair by feeding the young, but, when food is [in short supply] and other birds are not at the nest to witness exactly what the juveniles are doing, they consume the food themselves, sometimes even placing the food in the chicks' gaping beaks and then quickly swallowing it themselves. Such 'cheaters' show special enthusiasm for preening the young, and are apparently trying to impress their group members with their devotion" (pp. 224–225).

Pretending to be something one is not was apparently not invented in the age of Facebook!

But note in this last example how easy it is for researchers to slip from description to an interpretation of intentionality. According to these authors, there is a form of deliberate dupery going on here, the birds intending to fool their neighbors as to their good intentions and deeds. Such behavior could, however, be interpreted differently: the bird executes its usual helping behaviors (finding food and bringing it to the nest) but is so hungry that at the last minute it devours the food. In other words, no dissimulation may be intended here; the behavior just so happens to fool the other birds.

Lacan was quite interested in the question of faking, feigning, and dissimulation in the animal kingdom, insofar as he believed that it is the symbolic that allows for explicit forms of lying and pretending. In "Subversion of the Subject," he proposes that whereas animals may at times leave footprints in a certain direction to make potential predators think they went in that direction, even though they doubled back and went off in a different direction, they do not go the step further necessary to go beyond this level of feigning or faking and enter the world of signifiers. Here is what Lacan says there:

> Without the dimension [that the Other, specified as the locus of Speech] constitutes, the deceptiveness of Speech would be

indistinguishable from the feint, which, in fighting or sexual display, is nevertheless quite different. Deployed in imaginary capture, the feint is integrated into the play of approach and retreat [...]. Moreover, animals show that they are capable of such behavior when they are being hunted down; they manage to throw their pursuers off the scent by briefly going in one direction as a lure and then changing direction. This can go so far as to suggest on the part of game animals the nobility of honoring the parrying found in the hunt. But an animal does not *feign feigning*. It does not make tracks whose deceptiveness lies in getting them to be taken as false, when in fact they are true—that is, tracks that indicate the right trail. No more than it effaces its tracks, which would already be tantamount to making itself the subject of the signifier. (*Écrits*, p. 807; emphasis added)

Recall that for Lacan in Seminar IX, *Identification*, there are three stages in the constitution of the signifier: a disappearance, the erasing or effacing of the place where an object or track disappeared, and then a circling or marking of that same place (class given on January 24, 1962). It is the deliberate attempt to efface the trace of one's own passage somewhere that is, for Lacan, a sure sign of subjectivity, the kind of subjectivity brought into being by the signifying system. Smart criminals and conniving bankers are very adept at this, naturally; and according to Lacan, neurosis itself consists precisely in this attempt to erase one's own tracks, to dissimulate one's own involvement in situations, relationships, decisions, and so on. We can see this in the propensity among neurotics of all ilks to blind themselves to their own desires, their own motives in choices they make and actions they take, fantasies they have, pornography they watch, and so on. "What?" they protest, "I only watched that lesbian porn (or that aggressive prison porn) because an app started playing it automatically. I didn't go looking for it."

A further step in the kind of faking or feigning made possible by the signifying system is that of saying something that your interlocutor will believe is false when it is in fact true. Lacan refers to this as to "feign feigning." Imagine that your friends are going to a restaurant where the chef has a fabulous reputation and you know your friends like his cooking, but you secretly don't share their taste for it. So you say something that is likely to come off as a sarcastic remark in this context: you say you won't be joining them because the food stinks. Your friends will probably believe that it must be for some other reason that you are not going—you have a secret rendezvous you don't want to tell them about or you've maxed out your credit cards—but what you have said is in fact the real reason: you dislike the chef's cooking. Thus you have managed to dupe your friends and perhaps even spare their feelings by telling the truth!

In a recent real-life incident, a friend of mine, who is an inveterate jokester, had been spotted at a restaurant with a redhead no one knew anything about. Asked who she was, he gave various improbable answers, even suggesting at one point that she was his hairdresser, whereas he has exceedingly little hair to dress. Backed into a corner, he finally acquiesced and said he would tell me the truth, having first prepared the ground for me to take it as just one more lie: the supposed truth was that she was the director of the Michelin Restaurant Guide in France. As it turned out, she was! Perhaps it is not surprising that one of this friend's favorite personages is Talleyrand who once famously said, "Speech was given to man so that he could disguise his thought."

It is precisely this kind of feigned feigning that Lacan (*Écrits*, pp. 20 and 525) tries to bring out in Freud's discussion of the Jewish joke about the man going to Cracow. In "The Seminar on 'The Purloined Letter,'" Lacan writes:

> I shall confine my attention [...] to evoking the dialogue which seems to me to warrant its attribution as a Jewish joke due to the nakedness with which the relation between the signifier and speech appears in the entreaty which brings it to a head: "Why are you lying to me?" one character exclaims exasperatedly, "Yes, why are you lying to me by saying you're going to Cracow in order to make me believe you're going to Lemberg, when in reality you *are* going to Cracow?" (p. 20)[5]

Here the one speaker who is about to set off on a trip apparently knows that if he tells his interlocutor that he is going one place, his interlocutor is likely to believe he's going somewhere else—perhaps because his interlocutor never believes him or knows that the vast majority of the time the traveler lies to him. Here for some reason the interlocutor seems to know that the traveler *is* going to Cracow, which might lead us to wonder why he bothers to ask him where he's going in the first place (assuming he did ask)!

I think we can, in any case, sense the difference between this kind of exchange and the wagging dance of a bee returning to its hive to alert its fellow bees to a copious supply of pollen in a nearby field. We can hardly imagine its congeners wondering if the dancing bee is doing the particular dance it is doing in order to lure them into going off on a wild goose chase, there really being no pollen in that particular direction. Nor can we imagine its fellow bees thinking that this bee's dance is particularly cool and imitating it just for the sheer fun of it. Both of these would imply the kind of disjunction or hiatus between a sign system and the action it automatically triggers that is characteristic of signifying systems as opposed to simple sign systems.

An animal's world is characterized by all kinds of signs, signs being things that represent something to someone, to some being. The fact that a tiger marks a certain tree with its urine and/or anal gland secretions serves as a sign to another tiger that a potentially belligerent congener occupies this territory. Certain behaviors or expressions in the animal world have even taken on the value of signs in the sense that, if our ethologists are to be believed, they have taken on a more general meaning and can be used in contexts that are different from the ones in which they initially developed. For example, a dominant or alpha-male chimpanzee can give another chimpanzee who is lower on the dominance totem pole, so to speak, a bare-teeth grin which does not serve as an expression of fear but simply of friendliness and nonaggressive intentions: it "indicates that the sender is anxious to achieve a certain result, for instance to take over a desired resting place from a subordinate without fighting, or to establish peaceful contact with an attractive partner" (de Waal & Tyack, 2003, p. 285). Ethologists hypothesize that in these situations stereotypical expressions have become signs that are shortcuts for social interactions, in this case, ways of acknowledging the hierarchical relationship without testing or enforcing it.[6]

This could illustrate what Lacan says in his short article, "The Symbolic, the Imaginary, and the Real," included in a small volume entitled *On the Names-of-the-Father*:

> the elements of displaced instinctual behavior displayed by animals can give us a rough idea of a symbolic behavior. What is called symbolic behavior in animals is the fact that a displaced segment of such behavior takes on a socialized value and serves the animal group as a marker for a certain collective behavior. (Lacan, 2013, p. 12)

If such a stereotypical sign as a bare-teeth grin were then used by a monkey to lure another monkey into a false sense of security in order to take advantage of it, having thrown it off its guard, then we could perhaps begin to wonder whether monkeys had access to signifiers!

Much the same question—whether animals are largely confined to the imaginary register of images and signs, having no access to the symbolic per se—is reflected in Lacan's interest in whether or not animals can count. In plenty of bird and mammal species, parents seem quite aware when one of their sometimes numerous offspring is missing, but whether they can count as we do with an abstract notion of number seems far less likely: they recognize each of their offspring by its specific markings and odor, and can thus realize that one of them is missing without counting them. I won't go here into the many different opinions on the subject, but will simply cite a view by a historian of ethology, William Homan Thorpe:

> It was the outstanding feat of Otto Köhler and his pupils to produce the final but absolutely unequivocal results which showed that animals, especially birds, can "think unnamed numbers"—that is, they have a prelinguistic number sense; to some extent, they think without words. This is an achievement with which Otto Köhler's name will always be linked. (Thorpe, 1979, p. 113)

It is not entirely clear to me how anyone, much less bird brains, can "think unnamed numbers," but that certain animals may have a prelinguistic number sense at least does not strike me as nonsensical a priori. I believe that seals, dolphins, and monkeys have been able to identify certain groupings of objects as similar based on their number as opposed to anything else (such as shape or configuration), but I am not familiar enough with the research to make an educated judgment here.

The imaginary as dyadic relations

Speaking of numbers, Lacan makes it clear that whereas the imaginary is characterized by the number two, the symbolic is always characterized by at least three. As he says, again in the little volume entitled *On the Names-of-the-Father,*

THE MANY FACES OF THE IMAGINARY   93

> any analyzable relationship—that is, any relationship that is symbolically interpretable—is always inscribed in a three-term relationship. [...] This means that every two-term relationship is already more or less marked as imaginary in style. In order for a relationship to take on its symbolic value, the mediation of a third personage is necessary who, in relation to the subject, realizes the transcendent element thanks to which his relation to the object can be sustained at a certain distance. (Lacan, 2013, pp. 27–28)

I won't belabor the obvious importance Lacan places on the Other with a capital O as the third term between the two small others (a and a') present in the psychoanalytic setting. This third term is so crucial—whether it takes the form of the language the two parties speak to each other, the patient's history, or the larger cultural and political context—that without it clinicians are completely at sea in a relationship of one equal or semblable to another, having no compass to guide them in dealing with the patient's complaints except their own personal intuitions, or solutions that they themselves have found helpful in their own lives. The conveying of such personal intuitions or solutions amounts to nothing more than coaching.

The emphasis on this Other as the third party to every therapy relationship shows where Lacan diverges radically from so-called relational and intersubjective schools of psychoanalysis where there is no clear outside of the dyadic relationship subsisting between the two bodies that find themselves together in the consulting room. As Lacan puts it in "The Symbolic, the Imaginary, and the Real,"

> what is libidinally realizable between two subjects requires mediation. This is what gives its true value to the fact, asserted by psychoanalytic theory and demonstrated by experience, that nothing can be interpreted in the end—for that is what is at stake—except via Oedipus. (2013, pp. 27–28)

Oedipus obviously stands here for a tripartite structure, which Lacan renders more general with the broader notion of the symbolic order. This points already to the pointlessness of interpretation, strictly speaking, in analytic work with psychotics.

In the same lecture, Lacan adds that "a phenomenon is analyzable only if it represents something other than itself" (p. 15), which I believe we can understand, at least in part, as indicating that a bodily gesture or posture is only analyzable if it means something other than the fact that I just got bitten by a mosquito, for example, and that's why I'm scratching myself. It must have taken on some kind of symbolic, symptomatic meaning in order for it to be analyzable. It must involve some kind of message to the Other. It could be something as simple as "my parents won't let me touch my genitals in public, so I'll scratch some other part of my body in public in a way that is equally annoying to them but that they cannot justifiably complain about (because I manage to generate some kind of dermatitis that no one can diagnose)," or it could be far more displaced and disguised than that.

We find a noteworthy lack of such backhanded or cryptic messages to the Other in work with psychotics, where complaints about roommates, fellow workers, and bosses rarely if ever carry a second meaning, that of a complaint about the analyst. To insinuate to a psychotic that his speech may represent "something other than itself," that it may have a double meaning or a hidden or second intention, is to invite confusion. To insist that it means something other than itself is to begin to generate tension and perhaps even trigger paranoia. To repeatedly assert that a pipe is not a pipe and that a stomach ache means something more than an upset stomach may lead to a breaking off of the analysis and even a psychotic break.

As Lacan puts it in "Subversion of the Subject,"

> It is clear that Speech begins only with the passage from the feint to the order of the signifier, and that the signifier requires another locus—the locus of the Other, the Other as witness, the witness who is Other than any of the partners—for the Speech borne by the signifier to be able to lie, that is, to posit itself as Truth. (*Écrits*, p. 684)

Understanding is itself imaginary

Further development of the concept of the imaginary comes when Lacan formulates that to understand is itself imaginary, insofar as

A) One superimposes the image of something one thinks one already understands onto something one has before one that one does not understand, thereby reducing its specificity and in effect *misapprehending* it. In other words, understanding involves an attribution of meaning which is always and inevitably a short-circuiting of the situation at hand, a reduction of the complexity of the patient's world to a schematic interpretation that falls short of the goal.

B) Moreover, one imagines oneself as the kind of person who can understand (*on s'imagine—vous vous imaginez*, as he puts it in Seminar XXI, class given on November 13, 1973), and is proud of oneself for being understanding, intelligent, capable of helping others, and so on. To understand, whether it is the patient or the analyst who is doing the understanding, is always to congratulate oneself for having a certain handle or grasp on a situation, implying pleasure in a kind of mastery over one's behaviors or symptoms that is generally quite illusory. Indeed one of the most typical complaints on the part of patients is that, after numerous years of therapy, they understand why they behave as they do, but cannot stop behaving that way.

The reductionism inherent in the imaginary register

If, as a therapist, I work primarily in the imaginary register, I try to understand other people as if they were just like me, as if they thought the same way, or felt the same way about things, as I do. The imaginary involves looking at others and seeing myself, believing that others have the same motives, hang-ups, and anxieties I have. To the degree to which I consider them to have feelings, I think of them as just like mine. If I see a small child my own age fall down, I may well cry. (This is, we might say, our default mode as human beings, it requiring a considerable effort on our part to attempt to begin to see things from another's point of view. Parents and teachers devote strenuous efforts to get kids to try to put themselves in the shoes of people who are different from themselves.) When I am operating in the imaginary register, I compare everything others say with my own way of thinking: I believe that it makes sense when it conforms to my own way of thinking and operating in the world, and I believe that it does not make sense when it fails to conform to my own way of thinking and operating in the world. I take my own beliefs and feelings as the standard with which I compare everything else, and view all differing beliefs and feelings as stupid, unreasonable, or frankly incomprehensible.

This way of stating it, of course, already assumes that I am able to recognize that others' thoughts and beliefs differ from my own, but the fact is that when I am operating in the imaginary register I am likely to overlook the difference between our views and simply see and hear what I expect to see and hear, not what is there to be seen and heard. In the imaginary register, I am focused on what I believe the other person is saying and trying to say as opposed to what the other is actually saying. Insofar as I operate in the imaginary register, I cannot hear a slip of the tongue, because I immediately correct it in my mind with what *I* believe the other meant to say. I do not really need to hear the other speak, because I think I already know what she is going to say in advance, believing that I already comprehend her point of view even before I hear it.

Everything the other says or does from then on is interpreted in light of the conclusions I have already drawn; all of the other's actions are interpreted as fitting into an inflexible frame, none of her statements or actions being able to call the frame itself into question. In such cases, my frame has solidified into an "established paradigm" and, as we know from the history of science (see, for example, Kuhn, 1962), well-established paradigms often lead us to overlook facts that do not seem to fit into those paradigms or to cast doubt on or try to invalidate purported facts that might call those paradigms into question.

The imaginary register brings with it a frame or paradigm of just this sort, a paradigm based on the analyst's own particular, personal way of seeing the world. It thus involves a kind of constitutional blindness and deafness: blindness to difference, to anything radically Other that does not fit into the analyst's preconceived frame, and deafness to ambiguities in speech or slips of the tongue that impede comprehension, that might thwart the analyst's efforts to fit what she or he is hearing into a preexisting framework of meaning. This framework may, of course, include some material based on people other than the analyst him- or herself, for example friends and family members the analyst has known well, or the first few patients he or she encountered under supervision; but the impulse to understand will always lead to the same result: the reduction of the different to the same, the reduction of the patient's particularity to that of someone else the analyst has already known, if not loved.

In a word, the imaginary focuses on understanding, which virtually always involves jumping to conclusions about things we do not yet fully understand, if we ever do; and it focuses on meaning, which virtually always involves predigested, prefabricated meanings that derive from our own view of the world and not from our analysands' views of the world. Understanding is, in most cases, the endeavor to reduce something to what we already know (or think we already know),[7] an endeavor that in psychoanalysis we must refuse to the best of our ability. We would do well to begin with the premise that we most likely do not understand what our analysands are saying or what is going on for them, and to attempt to defer understanding for as long as possible, as Lacan (1993, chapter 1; Écrits, p. 471) often enjoins us to.

Nothing is harder than to grasp the specificity of what an individual analysand means by any particular formulation, often no matter how simple that formulation seems to be. An analysand of mine recently qualified some men he was interested in as "schmucks." Being from New York and thinking I knew the word meant "prick," I couldn't figure out what it was doing in the context, which was one of general admiration for these men. "Schmucks?" I reiterated. "Yeah, you know, 'regular guys,'" the analysand replied. If you think you know that a schmuck is a prick, think again: we never really speak the same language (Écrits, p. 282), and a prick is rarely the same thing for any two different people. If we believe it is, it is we analysts who fit Webster's definition of schmucks as "fools, oafs, or jerks."

Meaning is imaginary

The sketch I have provided here thus far of the imaginary is far from exhaustive, not including, as it does, many of Lacan's other glosses on the imaginary—related, for example, to narcissism, to the phallus as an image, and so on—but before ending today I would simply like to comment on one further discussion by Lacan of the imaginary, the one provided in 1973. At that time, Lacan returns to the notion that meaning is imaginary (which he had already formulated in Seminar III, p. 65, French pagination), saying, "The imaginary is what puts a stop to the deciphering [we do in analysis]; it is meaning" (Seminar XXI, class given on November 13, 1973). In other words, meaning crystallizes out from the deciphering of a dream at the point at which one stops the deciphering process—for example, stops associating to the various elements of the dream. Meaning in such instances is obviously provisional and can even be self-serving, insofar as putting an untimely end to the associating process may be designed to give an interpretation to the dream that is pleasing to oneself!

Obviously a stop must be put to the deciphering at some point, but whereas the deciphering itself partakes of the symbolic, the meaning that we arrive at or concoct is imaginary; simplistically stated, it provides a partial and possibly flattering image of oneself.

The imaginary as intuition

In that same seminar, Seminar XXI, Lacan relates the imaginary to intuition, and talks about how so many of our mathematical notions rely on visual images to illustrate them. Think, for example, of the notion of a one-to-one correspondence between elements in two sets, or of an isosceles or equilateral triangle, and you will see how important *seeing* or *visualizing* is to "understanding." Lacan seems to be particularly interested in knot theory precisely because we have such a difficult time imagining or illustrating on paper what a great many knots actually look like. Colloquially speaking, we could say that we have a hard time wrapping our heads around knots, finding them intuitively difficult to grasp, to distinguish from each other, and so on. There is always, Lacan says, "a share of intuition in what mathematicians begin with."

Knot theory requires us to at least attempt to dispense with intuition. So if you can find precious little to like in Lacan's seemingly endless discussions of knots in the 1970s, I would suggest that his attempt to get psychoanalysts to try to dispense with intuition at least every now and again is an exceedingly important antidote to contemporary trends in psychotherapy and psychoanalysis.

When Lacan discusses consistency, he says that we tend to take the body as a model for understanding the rest of the universe (as in phenomenological psychology, where this is celebrated, not deconstructed), the body being understood largely on the basis of our images of it; this is not the case in knot theory. The body is thus the source or foundation of a great deal of what we refer to as "intuition." When we try to understand reality in terms of our bodies, with their front/back, top/bottom, right/left, and inside/outside configurations, we often run into trouble quickly, whether we are trying to grasp the so-called heavenly bodies or subatomic particles.

Note that even though Lacan devotes considerable effort in Seminar XXI to claiming that, unlike what people had concluded about his teaching up until then—namely, that the symbolic was of far greater importance than the imaginary—actually all three registers are of equal importance, we nevertheless find him putting down intuition and extolling the virtues of the real. As he says there, "Models have recourse to the pure imaginary, whereas knots have recourse to the real and take on their value from the fact that they have no less scope in the mental realm than in reality [or: than the real does, *dans le mental que le Réel*], even if the mental realm is imaginary." Indeed, we might almost argue that, for Lacan in the 1970s, it is no longer the symbolic that takes precedence over the imaginary, but the real that takes precedence over both the imaginary and the symbolic.

I will leave you with a final quote from 1973:

> The imaginary is always an intuition of what must be symbolized. As I just said, it is something to be chewed or mulled over, as they say. Indeed, it is a vague jouissance. Human beings get off on more widely varied things than you think, even if they are limited by something related to the body, to the human body. (Seminar XXI, class given on November 13, 1973)

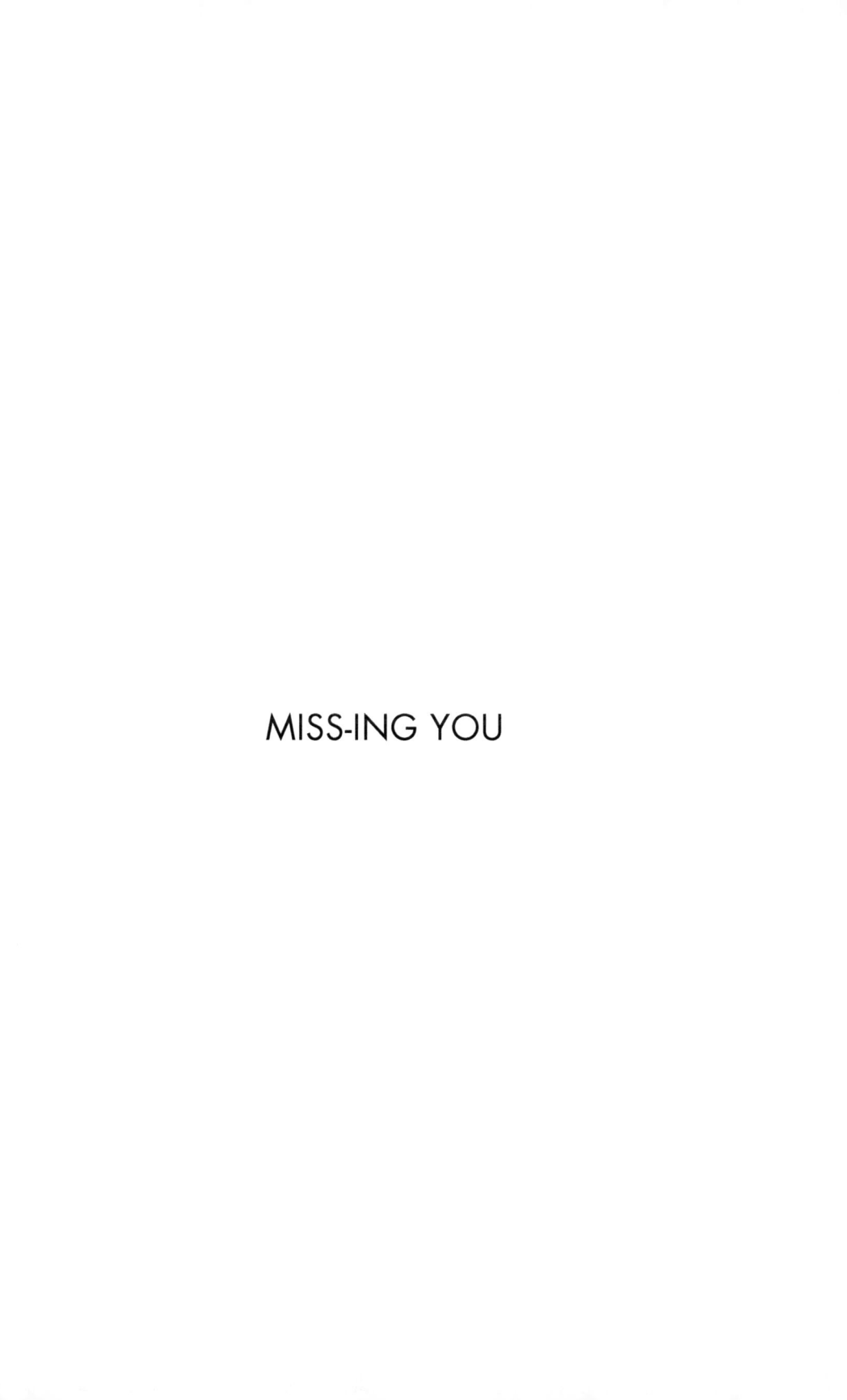

CHAPTER 4

Love, warts and all

(This talk was given, at the invitation of Ivan Ward, at the Freud Museum in London, as a part of the "Freud Today, Freud Tomorrow" conference on September 24–25, 2016.)

> *Your own symptoms are the only thing about you, or about anyone else, that are of interest.*[1]
>
> —Lacan (Seminar XXIII, p. 165)

I would like to begin by thanking Ivan Ward for inviting me today, and thank you all for coming.[2] Ivan indicated that I could talk about whatever was foremost in my mind at that time, and although I was already well into writing an introduction to Freud's work specifically designed for practicing clinicians, I was still thinking a good deal about Freud's and Lacan's work on love, having spent the prior year writing a book on the topic, entitled *Lacan on Love* (Fink, 2016; and let the record show that I wanted to entitle it "Love is giving what you don't have," but my editor rejected that title as overly obscure). Hence my talk today, which only indirectly touches on Freud's notions of love when I turn to the topic of transference and transference love.

I discussed transference love at some length in *Fundamentals of Psychoanalytic Technique* (Fink, 2007), where I began the task of comparing and contrasting Lacanian versus other psychoanalytic schools' notions of transference. That is no easy task insofar as each school has developed its own oftentimes idiosyncratic vocabulary, and inasmuch as each school uses the same words to mean different things. This led what was initially planned to be a rather short chapter to become by far the longest chapter in the book. I will continue this exploration of transference to at least a small degree this morning, approaching it from the direction of love as Lacan discusses it in Seminar VIII.

I will pick up on a couple of points in that Seminar that I commented on only briefly in *Lacan on Love*, comments that seem to have been confusing and/or unconvincing to certain readers who have contacted me, and that thus perhaps require elucidation.

Certain facets of Lacan's account of love are by now fairly well known, at least I hope they are. In particular, I suspect that many of you are familiar with the following notion, which I will paraphrase from Lacan's commentary late in Seminar VIII on Paul Claudel:

> What is asked of us in love is not our *poros*, our resources, our spiritual richness, our overabundance, or even, as Claudel puts it, our joy; rather, what is asked of us is precisely what we do not have. (p. 308)

When we love, it is not what we have and what it is thus easy for us to give that we must offer our beloved (as Lacan says, "Giving what you have is throwing a party [*c'est la fête*], not love" (p. 357); what we must offer our beloved is, rather, what we don't have, what we feel lacking in, and are thus most loath to avow and hand over. What we must convey to our beloved is our sense that we are incomplete, lacking in something, and searching for something; this leads our beloved to feel that we are exposing to him or her our lack, our deepest vulnerability—the very thing that most of us spend so much time and energy hiding from the world. It is by making this admission, which for many (perhaps above all for those who are quite obsessive) is quite difficult to make, that our beloved is likely to feel most loved by us.

I attempted, in *Lacan on Love*, to extend this notion by saying that it is not simply that our beloved feels most loved when we express this lack to him or her; we feel most loved when we ourselves feel appreciated not merely for what we have (our possessions, our good qualities, and so on); we ourselves feel most loved when we feel appreciated for our lack, our faults and failings, our defects—in a word, when we feel loved for what *we* do not have. To put it in more psychoanalytic terms, perhaps, we feel most loved when we are loved for being split subjects who do not know what we are saying or doing at times, when we are loved for our unconscious, our symptoms, our fundamental fantasy even. We do not feel most loved when we are loved for the same things or qualities that plenty of other people have, whether that be intelligence, power, money, a certain kind of physical stature, facial bone structure, hair color, eye color, or what have you. We want to be loved for what makes us *different* from everyone else, and what essentially makes us different is our unconscious, our symptoms, and our jouissance—these constitute our "subjective difference" from other people.

Everything else about us is subject to comparison with other people on a scale of more or less; but we sense, it seems to me, that our unconscious is unique. Even if many people have some of the same symptoms, and even if a certain number of people perhaps share some facets of our fundamental fantasy, we—or at least many of us, and perhaps especially those who have undergone an analysis—sense that what makes us uniquely us is our unconscious and our own specific way of enjoying ourselves, our own singular way of experiencing jouissance.

Some of us are not unaware that what we get off on is unpalatable if not downright disgusting to many potential partners, and that our failings, flaws, symptoms, slips, and bungled actions may lead plenty of people to steer clear of us. But that does not stop us from feeling most accepted when our so-called defects do not lead our partners to avoid us, even if we ourselves do not accept those defects and wish to find a way to get rid of them—that is, even if we are conflicted about them and prefer not to see them as part and parcel of our selves.

People are inclined to formulate such acceptance by saying that such partners love us "in spite of" our faults, our weaknesses, and our neuroses. In the vernacular, they are said to love us "warts and all." (This expression is said by some to have first been uttered by Oliver Cromwell when asking the painter Sir Peter Lely to paint a portrait of him as he truly was, rather than make him look better than he was in real life, as was typical at the time.)[3]

In *Lacan on Love*, I attempted to take this another step further by saying that we want to be loved not merely *in spite of* our warts, but indeed *because of* our warts, because of our defects. Our "warts" go right to the core of us far more than all the other features that most people can see, far more than what we are willing to show most people. We don't want to feel that our warts are things that are subtracted from our supposed qualities, making us a little bit or perhaps even a lot less loved than we might otherwise be by our partner, especially given that our current qualities may not last forever: we may begin losing our hair or it may turn gray, our intelligence may dim to some degree, our physical stature may change over the course of time, and so on. As our qualities wane, will our warts begin to outweigh them? If so, the love we receive from our beloved will appear increasingly precarious, as it is conditional upon the ability of our qualities to overshadow our faults, conditional upon the balance sheet of our assets and liabilities.

One of my analysands admitted to me that he had a bad habit, as he called it, of adopting what one of his partners dubbed a "clinical gaze": even as he was making love to them, he would focus on small physical anomalies they had, like bumps on their skin or stretch marks, and on their smell to which he was particularly attuned. A couple of the women with whom he was involved over the years would notice him dwelling on these little particularities, and felt very much unloved by this kind of attention. He would offhandedly joke about their imperfections, in the naïve belief that he could convince them that he found these features funny or endearing, whereas in fact they turned him off and sometimes even disgusted him. The more he tried to laugh it off, the more he dug his own grave, so to speak, his partners apparently not wishing to be loved because their qualities outweighed their imperfections: they wanted to be loved lock, stock, and barrel.

Thus, although we may be conflicted about what we perceive to be our imperfections—insofar as we try to get rid of some of them through diet, exercise, medical treatments, plastic surgery, and sometimes even psychoanalysis—we ourselves at least at some level want to be loved *for* our warts, not in spite of them.

Something that seems to me to be less well understood by many of Lacan's readers than the idea that to love is to give what we do not have is the notion that *what we love in our beloved is what our beloved does not have*. Lacan explicitly states this in Seminar IV: "What we love when we love is what is truly beyond the subject: it is literally what he doesn't have" (p. 128).[4] If we are to truly love, what we must love in our beloved is his or her lack, failings, faults, slips, bungled actions—in a word, his or her unconscious and all that the unconscious brings with it, including symptoms and specific ways of getting off.[5]

Now that is a very tall order! But it is in fact no more than the corollary of what we ourselves want, insofar as we want to be loved *for* our warts, because of our warts.

To make such a discussion perhaps easier to grasp, let us consider a real life example that involves the register of *friendship*, not that of a love relationship per se. Let us consider a friend of mine who has some good qualities (I'll call them X, Y, and Z) and some not-so-good characteristics (P, Q, and R). On the good qualities side, we have someone who:

X: Has amazing taste in wine and fine cuisine and extensive knowledge of them.
Y: Is very quick witted and makes jokes and snappy comebacks a mile a minute, keeping me in stitches.
Z: Gives money to worthy charitable causes.

On the bad characteristics side, we have a guy who:

P: Is clueless as to what it means to be friends, not just with me but with most people, at least as far as I can tell, and has no idea how to maintain and cultivate a relationship. Instead of calling, or writing about something personal that actually took some thinking on his part about me, his correspondent, he sends out impersonal group emails full of cartoons and links to vaguely amusing articles. Worse still, he almost never returns invitations to parties or dinners, even though he seems happy to come when invited.
Q: He may be somewhat immoral in his business dealings.
R: His personal rule of thumb regarding people is "never forgive, never forget."

Now I'm going to pretend that he is your friend, not mine, and I'm going to pretend, moreover, that you continue to see this bloke. Shall we say that you do so because you feel his good traits outweigh his bad ones? Shall we say, in other words, that you engage in some sort of calculation, adding up the good, subtracting the bad, and as long as he stays in the black—as long as something remains in the plus column—you are still willing to see him? This could be true for some of you, the result being that the day the total comes out in the red (that is, negative), you write him off as a pure and simple loss; the day he stops being so witty or stops contributing to charities you approve of, you drop him.

Others, perhaps those with something of a psychological bent, might excuse his flaws on the basis of his upbringing and shattered family life, his parents having divorced early and his mother having had to struggle to raise her children alone. In other words, others of you might cut him some slack. How much slack? An infinite amount? That seems rather unlikely …

What could possibly keep you wanting to maintain a one-sided friendship with such a person? Love, perhaps. How's that? Is it that love allows you to *ignore* the faults or flaws that you find in his character traits to the point of overlooking them completely, or does it go further still? Does it go so far as to allow you—who are, after all, divided subjects in your own right, who are not all of one mind about the vast majority of things—to see P, Q, and R as worthy of love, not scorn?

Maybe there is something in you that would secretly like to treat people as badly or one-sidedly as he does, to be as asocial or flaunt conventions like he does, and to only have people over when you really want to instead of kowtowing to the rules of social interaction that require you to return invitations. Perhaps, too, you would like to stop feeling that you have to forgive and forget everyone's slights and lack of consideration towards you—it perhaps seeming to you that you are the only one who forgives, everyone else remembering each and every one of your oversights, outbursts, and peccadillos. Perhaps it seems that it would be nice to be able to be more extreme at times, to just go with the way you really feel like acting, instead of tempering your reactions and moderating your criticism, instead of always wrestling with yourself and yielding to your conscience. At times we might consider such extreme and uncompromising attitudes praiseworthy and envy those who seem to us to have them, even if they are the exact opposite of attitudes we try to cultivate in ourselves—exact opposites so often being indicative of the clash between conscious and unconscious, as Freud tells us in his case study of Dora: "Opposite thoughts are always closely connected with each other and are often paired in such a way that *the one thought is excessively, intensely conscious while its opposite is repressed and unconscious*" (SE VII, p. 55). Perhaps you consciously hate his flaunting of conventions, but unconsciously love and admire it!

And maybe there is some part of you that gets a bit of a thrill or *frisson* out of his being somewhat on the edge morally when it comes to the rules of business and taxation. Maybe you get a big kick out of movies about heists, jewel thieves, and bank robbers, and identify with such characters when you see or hear about them in action, and perhaps even secretly fantasize about being one yourself someday, even if you probably would never actually allow yourself to do so.

In other words, those of you who continue to see this guy—even though you may occasionally or even often wonder why you keep doing so, or kick yourself when his bad behavior gets on your nerves ("Why did I invite him over again?")—may well have ended up loving his warts. In spite of all your conscious deliberations about this guy's "unfrequentability" as they say in French (*il est infréquentable*), and his "untakeoutability" (*insortable*), as they also say in French, you have grown to love his more dubious qualities. You now love even those things about him, even if your love for them remains unconscious—that is, even if you continue to tell yourself and everyone else that you hate them.

Hopefully the transition from this less than fictional example in the realm of friendship—that I have ungraciously and unceremoniously foisted upon you rather than take full responsibility for it myself—to other examples in the realm of love relationships will strike you as smooth and seamless.

In *Lacan on Love*, I wrote:

> Can we, after all, love someone who seems to us to be perfect, someone who seems to us to *have* everything? Isn't it often the case that although we may be fascinated or captivated by someone who appears to have only good qualities, we only begin to love him or her from the moment we suspect that he or she is somewhat (if not deeply) unhappy, quite clueless about something, rather awkward, clumsy, or helpless? Isn't it in his or her nonmastery or incompleteness that we see a possible place for ourselves in his or her affections—that is, that we glimpse the possibility that we may be able to do something for that person, be something to that person? In this sense, we perhaps love *not* what they have, but what they do not have. (2016, p. 41)

In other words, I formulated our love for the other's lack, failings, or faults only in terms of our search to play an important role in that person's life—in other words, in terms of a narcissistic project to have a privileged place in that person's affections, thereby winning ourselves love in the process. Here I am trying to suggest that it is perhaps more complicated than that.

Note that Lacan himself says something similar to what I am saying here in discussing Freud's case of the "young homosexual woman" (SE XVIII, pp. 147–172), where he suggests that the young woman in question wanted to show her father what it really means to love someone:

> [What she shows him] in her exalted love for her lady is, as Freud tells us, the exact model of absolutely altruistic love, thoroughly gratuitous love […]. What she demonstrates to her father is how one can love someone, not only for what that person has but for what that person does not have. (Seminar IV, pp. 144–145)[6]

The woman she loved (in what Freud characterized as the manner of a knight for his lady in courtly love times) did not have very much: she did not have high social status, was apparently not wealthy, had no family of her own, and thus obviously did not have what he refers to as the phallus. The young homosexual woman seems to have felt that her father believed that only those who *had* something were worthy of love (perhaps they even had to have a lot, even if only potentially, like someone who could provide a legitimate heir to the family name), and she set out to show him *how one goes about loving someone for what she does not have*, and to give her what she herself did not have (herself as a phallus, Lacan says).[7]

The use and abuse of countertransference

Now what might be the implications of such notions of love for the analytic setting? Freud early on introduced the notion of "transference love," and eventually indicated that there was no theoretical difference between transference love and ordinary love. The same could obviously be said of "countertransference love," to coin a phrase. In other words, both transference love and countertransference love involve the same stakes as romantic or what is sometimes referred to as affectionate or companionate love. And by extension, we might hypothesize that transference hate and countertransference hate, which are the flip side of transference love and countertransference love and are thus intimately related to them, involve the same stakes as hatred as it appears in everyday life.

As a supervisor of a wide variety of clinicians, I hear quite a lot about countertransference love and hate, and thus I would like to return to the topic of countertransference, which, as many of you are probably aware, Lacan defined already in 1951 as arising from the analyst's own problems. As he put it, countertransference is "the sum total of the analyst's biases, passions, and difficulties, or even of his inadequate information, at any given moment in the dialectical process" of analysis (*Écrits*, p. 225). In a word, Lacan theorized *countertransference as arising from a mistake analysts make—usually unwittingly—in the way they position themselves in the analyses they conduct*. In Lacan's view, analysts, by reviewing cases alone and/or in conjunction with a supervisor, must figure out how to reposition themselves in the analysis such that countertransference is at least significantly allayed.

Let me briefly recall to mind a couple of instances in which Freud situated himself problematically in his own analytic practice.

I'll start with the case of the Rat Man, whose real name was Ernst Langer.[8] In one of his very first sessions, Langer began to tell Freud about the severe crisis that started during the military maneuvers he was part of in August 1907. Langer mentioned Captain Nemeczek (Freud, 2000, p. 55), "the cruel captain" as Freud dubbed him, whose story about the form of torture involving rats had such a big impact on him. But at one point in the story, the following happened, according to Freud:

> The patient broke off, got up from the sofa, and begged me to spare him the recital of the details. *I assured him that I myself had no taste whatsoever for cruelty, and certainly had no desire to torment him*, but that naturally *I could not grant him something that was beyond my power*. He might just as well ask me to give him the sun and the moon. The overcoming of resistances was *the law of psychoanalytic treatment*, and on no consideration could be dispensed with. [...] I went on to say that I would do all I could, nevertheless, to guess the full meaning of any hints he gave me. (SE X, p. 166; my emphasis)

Freud's first "guess" involved impalement and his second guess the anus. One of the immediate results of Freud's insistence on knowing what the patient was finding it so difficult to say aloud was that Langer began calling Freud "Captain" during the very same session (SE X, p. 169), presumably having found rather cruel Freud's insistence on his overcoming his resistance so early on in the treatment! Freud's disclaimer—"I assure you, I have no taste for cruelty"—was belied by his insistence, proving itself to be a typically untrustworthy denial or negation (Freud, 2000, p. 43). The patient was undoubtedly aware that Freud could have waited a week or a month before learning the exact nature of the torture, and that the supposed "law" to which Freud professed to be submitting was actually a law of his own making (Langer had, after all, read some of Freud's writings prior to beginning analysis with him).

To be generous, I believe we can say that Freud did not deliberately try to get himself associated with the cruel captain by the Rat Man, but he nevertheless made a mistake in positioning himself in the analysis by insisting that the patient make certain revelations in the very first sessions. This was part of Freud's long-standing countertransferential *passion for everything to come out as quickly as possible*, certainly not in the patient's own good time, a passion he seems to have expressed with most if not all of his patients right up until the end of his work as a practitioner. It is not clear that Freud was ever able to completely overcome this initial mistake in his positioning with Langer.

Freud's mistake in the case of Dora, whose real name was Ida Bauer, was far worse, I would argue, he having overly identified early on in the analysis with Herr K as a still young, good-looking man whom Freud believed would actually be a good catch and a good match for Bauer. He believed this based on his own ideas, prejudices, and only partial information about Herr K (which is all we ever have as analysts and which is why we should not take sides or give advice!); recall that Freud had met Herr K on at least one occasion. Freud foolishly concluded that Herr K had in good faith propositioned Bauer by the lake the day she ended up slapping him and believed that Herr K intended to divorce his wife and marry Bauer. This was belied by Bauer's revelation at the very end of her work with Freud that Herr K had made a very similar proposal (using some of the exact same words) to his children's governess, whom he had seduced and then quickly dumped.

Imprudently jumping to conclusions about Herr K, Freud ended up situating himself in the analysis with Bauer at least partly as a suitor for her affections, which perhaps led him to attempt to come up with what he considered to be brilliant interpretations of her dreams and of her every gesture and bodily movement so that she would admire and perhaps even love him for them. As we know, all that brilliance was wasted—his interpretations either simply irked her or, worse still, rolled off her like water off a duck's back, leaving her cold. His attempt to be loved by her for what he *had*—mountains of interpretations—seems to have failed miserably.

The other facet of Freud's positioning of himself in the analysis was as more of a father figure or father confessor who insisted upon her confessing everything to him *in full* as early on in the treatment as possible so that he could single-handedly resolve her symptoms, instead of helping her come to terms with her own symptoms.

Freud purportedly admitted the following to Abraham Kardiner (1977) in the 1920s:

> I have several handicaps that disqualify me as a great analyst. One of them is that I am too much the father. Second, I am much too occupied with theoretical problems all the time, so that whenever I get occasion, I am working on my own theoretical problems, rather than paying attention to the therapeutic problems. Third, I have no patience in keeping [patients] for a long time. I tire of them, and I want to spread my influence. (pp. 68–69)

It is not difficult to see how all three of these "handicaps" played a role in his work with Bauer twenty years earlier, he having (1) overly identified with other father figures in the case; (2) subordinated the individual work with her to the attempt to find clinical proof of the theory of dream interpretation he had just published in *The Interpretation of Dreams*; and (3) wanted to get everything out into the open as quickly as possible and clear everything up right away, rather than giving Bauer time to come to trust him, open up, and question and interpret things herself, which she at least occasionally appears to have done, short as their work together was.

All three of these handicaps were obviously part and parcel of Freud's countertransference and probably to some degree affected *all* of the analyses he ever conducted. This is not to say that we contemporary analysts are free from biases, passions, and inadequate information ourselves!

In any case, working in a vacuum without the help of a supervisor who might have been able to detect his over-involvement in the Dora case right from the first, Freud never seems to have realized that he had mispositioned himself in the analysis. Even at the very end, when he was writing up the case, he seems not to have seen that he himself identified with Herr K, but instead believed that it was Bauer alone who associated him with Herr K—which she probably did to some small extent just because they were both men of a certain age and both smokers (but note that it was Freud himself who pointed this latter out to her, thereby highlighting their similarity). Freud was convinced that Bauer had figuratively slapped him in the face when she broke off the treatment with him, like she had literally slapped Herr K at the lake. Freud unwittingly ended up acting just like Herr K did, when Herr K did not openly and formally propose marriage to Bauer after the slap: rather than honorably entreating Bauer to continue the analysis after she announced she'd be leaving, Freud let her go, felt embittered, and blamed much of the failure of the analysis on her. In a word, he attributed to her transference the problematic positioning that constituted his own countertransference. Allow me to repeat that: *he attributed to her transference the problematic positioning that constituted his own countertransference.*

Now how common is that?! Isn't that what therapists do all the time these days? A broad swath of contemporary psychoanalysts has adopted the notion that the patient is responsible for virtually everything the analyst is thinking, feeling, daydreaming about, annoyed by, or distracted by during sessions and even between sessions, because patients are theorized to project all kinds of things *into* their analysts, which thus get "inside" their analysts through no doing of their own.

If the analyst falls asleep, the patient is making the analyst fall asleep either deliberately or by "putting sleepiness into the air" (this is the exact phrase the analyst of a friend of mine used to make his falling asleep her fault). If the analyst suddenly notices his stomach is gurgling, the patient must have done something to upset his stomach. If the analyst begins worrying about his own health, like Thomas Ogden (1994) did with a patient he calls Mrs. B, and suffers from a "somatic delusion" in the course of the session instead of listening to his patient, his patient must be resenting him and wanting him dead just like she wanted her own father dead (pp. 477–483). If the analyst is feeling pressured to interpret something or come up with a solution to some particular problem, the patient must be pressuring him to give answers.[9]

This new theoretical perspective goes by a variety of names— relational psychoanalysis, interpersonal psychoanalysis, intersubjectivity, and Kleinian/Bionian psychoanalysis, all of which seem to rely heavily on the notion of projective identification.[10] I will not attempt to do justice here to the differences among them, my interest being in commenting on what all of them, in my view, attempt to accomplish. Some analysts in these different modern schools of analysis profess to pay attention to the countertransference, without ever directly revealing it to the analysand, others reveal it at times, others still use it systematically, and most of them seem to be on the constant lookout for any and every possible allusion in the analysand's discourse to how the analysand thinks the analyst is reacting to him or feeling about what he says, and these so-called allusions are at times more than just a little far-fetched!

Unfairly lumping all of these schools of psychoanalysis together, and speaking quite cynically, I would suggest that this new theoretical perspective accomplishes at least three things (whether it was designed to accomplish them or not is an open question):

1) It places the blame for the analyst's problematic positioning in the analysis on the patient. If I seem to be finding myself in a bind in my work with a patient, it is not my fault but rather the patient's. If I am furious at a patient for something, this is not owing to my own neuroses, passions, inadequate information, or biases, but rather to the patient's. As analysts we should, it seems to me, always be extremely suspicious of such convenient explanations that seem to shore up our analytic ego-ideal, allowing us to think that we are, after all, and notwithstanding appearances to the contrary, good, caring, intelligent, helpful people who don't have a mean streak or a resentful bone in our whole bodies.

2) This new theory also seems designed to allow us to turn something that, earlier in the history of psychoanalysis, was viewed as a flaw or defect in the analyst into a virtue. Analysts' supposed ability to sense all kinds of things that are being put or projected into them by their analysands is now thought to manifest extraordinary sensitivity on their part! They must be incredibly attuned to their patients if they are able to feel or pick up on all of those things. Some may find what I am saying here flippant, but I am inclined to think that analysts who are enamored of the more or less direct use of countertransference in their work with patients are attempting to make a virtue of a failing. Analysands here take most, if not all, of the blame (for upsetting or destructive projections, for example) and analysts take most, if not all, of the credit (for exquisite sensitivity and gruelingly emotional work).

3) Third, this new theory, insofar as it leads to a form of practice in which the analyst's reactions, feelings, and reveries take center stage (and this is admittedly the case more for certain analysts than for others), seems to allow those analysts who perhaps felt that their daily work was not enough *about them* to make it more about them; it seems to offer a solution to those who felt their work with analysands required too much self-denial or demanded that they put themselves aside to a degree that they found difficult to sustain. Such analysts are perhaps quite pleased to be able to embrace a theory of the analytic situation that allows them to regularly talk about how they themselves think and feel to their analysands.

Let me illustrate how this new perspective tries to turn a defect or liability into a virtue by briefly commenting on an article by a well-known American psychoanalyst by the name of Owen Renik, "Analytic Interaction: Conceptualizing Technique in Light of the Analyst's Irreducible Subjectivity." It was given pride of place in Stephen A. Mitchell and Lewis Aron's 1999 collection entitled *Relational Psychoanalysis: The Emergence of a Tradition*, which, as you may know, grew into a multi-volume series of 500-page books compiling those articles considered to represent the many facets of the contemporary relational/intersubjective movements. Renik, a defining figure within these movements, makes his positions very clear, and I will quote some of them at length here:

> Instead of saying that it is *difficult* for an analyst to *maintain* a position in which his or her analytic activity objectively focuses on the patient's inner reality, I would say that it is *impossible* for an analyst to be in that position *even for an instant*: since we are constantly acting in the analytic situation on the basis of personal motivations of which we cannot be aware until after the fact, our technique, listening included, is inescapably subjective. (1999, p. 414)

A page later, he adds,

> We are always completely personally involved in our judgments and decisions, and it is precisely at those moments when we believe that we are able to be objective-as-opposed-to-subjective that we are in the greatest danger of self-deception and departure from sound methodology. (p. 415)

Most of us would, I suspect, agree that we analysts are not merely objective observers or listeners; yet we strive, or at least I hope we do, to pay very close attention to the patient's discourse, as opposed to what Renik calls the "patient's inner reality," whatever that may be. Note that many analysts today talk about the "patient's inner reality" as though it were something that were immediately accessible to the analyst, instead of being mediated by the patient's speech. It is our attention to the patient's speech that sets limits to the degree to which what we do and say is about us as opposed to about the patient. It is the patient's speech that we can record on paper and share with colleagues, even if we cannot easily convey the tone of voice and cadence with which that speech is uttered; but, with the patient's permission, we can even electronically record it, allowing a group of analysts to all work from the same material. This attention to the patient's speech is perhaps what sets Lacanians apart from other contemporary practitioners.

Although Renik admits that "we should not impose our truths, whether or not theory laden; we should maintain our focus on the patient's inner reality," in his view, "Again and again, we fail to adhere to these precepts. *Despite our best intentions, we seem to have a fundamental disinclination to maintaining these positions*" (p. 414). And there begins his attempt to bring to bear all the things analysts are thinking about and feeling when they are *not* listening to their patients, to bring all of that to bear on the analysis in some sort of supposedly useful way.

It seems to me that the attempt to turn a failing into a virtue is most apparent here. A "fundamental disinclination" to do what our theory of practice tells us to do would presumably be a reason to go back into analysis or begin supervision with a new supervisor. Instead, this "disinclination" to focus on the patient seems to have become reason enough to call into question our entire theory and practice! For someone like Renik, such a disinclination is no longer problematic; rather, it is the very theory that would have us believe that we *should* focus on the patient and must thus obviously become able to focus on the patient that is questionable. The theory itself is impugned as faulty and must be jettisoned because of certain analysts' "fundamental disinclination" to focus on what the patient is saying.

In a word, our theory of practice must be wrong if we are unable to practice as the theory says we should. We need not call ourselves into question, we need not wonder whether perhaps we might benefit from a new stint of analysis, we need not consider this to be a failing of our own, we need not wonder if we are perhaps not cut out for this one of the three impossible professions. There are, in Renik's view, enough analysts out there who feel this way to prove that this is "the new normal," so to speak; objectivity is passé, if there ever was such a thing, and there is no reason for us to continue to strive for it.

What then does the analyst end up relying upon? According to Renik, the analyst relies on "His *intuitive understanding* of the patient's state of mind and character" (p. 416; my emphasis).[11] I won't comment here on "understanding" as I recently published a two-volume collection of papers entitled *Against Understanding*. The emphasis or not on understanding constitutes one of the major differences between traditional forms of psychoanalysis and most Lacanian forms, Lacanians tending to aim at something beyond understanding.

Instead, let me raise the question "What is intuition?" "Intuition" is nothing but a sense one has or a guess one makes that is based on unarticulated, unexamined notions that one has assimilated in the course of one's lifetime, and that is based on commonly heard phrases about life and people in our culture. So-called intuition is shaped by everything one has heard and read growing up, much of which is informed by a mishmash of psychological theories, whether espoused by novelists, poets, filmmakers, songwriters, talk-show hosts, or parents and friends. It seems to me that once recourse is had to the analyst's "intuition," the patient's speech and psychoanalytic theory go out the window in one fell swoop. If intuition in the psychoanalytic setting is considered to be something only the most seasoned analysts have, then it is presumably based on long experience working with analysands of different kinds, and should, in theory, be articulable, not merely gestured toward as a special gift that only certain analysts possess (see *Écrits*, p. 210).

Renik concludes his paper on "the analyst's irreducible subjectivity" with the following: "It has been my purpose to propose that we aim toward a revision in our basic theory of technique that will make it unnecessary for us to ask ourselves, in vain, not to be passionately and irrationally involved in our everyday clinical work" (1999, p. 421). How can we respond to such a conclusion other than by saying *"Dude!"* (Owen Renik is, after all, from the West Coast) or *"Incroyable!"*

Intuition is not the only thing the analyst is said to be able to rely on, according to theoreticians and practitioners of this new tendency in psychoanalysis; there is also what Thomas Ogden (1994) has dubbed the "analytic third." The analytic third in no wise transcends what

Lacan calls the imaginary register, however; indeed, it might well be equated with the "imaginary axis" itself (Ogden himself admits that it is not "third" in Lacan's sense of the symbolic that interrupts the dyadic relation; p. 464). Christopher Bollas (1983) refers instead to what he calls "the Other patient," who turns out to be the analyst himself, but who is supposed to be the patient as we find him or her "within" the analyst! This clearly has nothing to do with Lacan's symbolic Other and seems to me to verge on a form of mysticism.

What is it about what goes on in psychoanalysis that makes it so much more difficult for many contemporary practitioners to focus on what provides whatever bit of objectivity we can and do have in psychoanalysis—namely, what the patient actually says (even if we might not all hear what the patient says in exactly the same way)—than it is for medical doctors, nurses, dentists, lawyers, accountants, and other service providers to focus on what provides the objectivity they have in their own fields? Doctors who prescribe a course of treatment that has little if any connection to what are known as best practices, the standard of care, or what the current research in their field supposedly shows (even if it eventually turns out to be false) are generally considered negligent. Their judgment may at times be clouded by their interest in a specific patient, they being overly worked up because of some personal connection between the patient and themselves. But for the most part, doctors, like dentists, lawyers, accountants, plumbers, roofers, car mechanics, and so on, rely quite easily on the more or less well-established knowledge in their fields and its relevance to the case at hand. All such practitioners may, at times, deviate from what they would otherwise do if they were not personally involved with the person whose divorce they are handling or whose tax return they are preparing. They probably don't run away to Brazil with every man who shows up at their office seeking a divorce, or steal all the money of every woman who turns to them for their accounting services, but instead try to advise them and guide them based on the client's wishes (even if unrealistic and/or self-contradictory) and a more or less thorough knowledge of the legal system, the tax code, the judge who they are likely to appear before if there will be a court appearance, and so on. Why is it that we can expect at least some degree of objectivity from our car mechanic (even if some are obviously far sharper than others), but not from our psychoanalyst?

Surely it must have something to do with the personal and emotionally laden nature of the material that gets discussed in the consulting room; yet some such personal and emotionally laden material also gets discussed in physicians' and lawyers' offices, not to mention those of private investigators. For some reason we have reached a point in history where we no longer expect psychoanalysts—who have all been through a relatively long training program and an at least somewhat long training analysis—to base what they do in the analytic setting on anything other than intuition, or on their feelings (feelings which they attempt to formulate as echoing the patient's feelings or even as reflecting the feelings the patient isn't feeling but would be feeling if only he were in touch with his feelings!). What sense can we possibly make of that?

Before addressing such an intractable question (which may arise owing to the inadequacies of contemporary psychoanalytic training, where it is said people often do their first analysis for the school, and, it having been more or less useless, do a second one for themselves, assuming they can afford to and still have the will to), let us consider the sorts of psychoanalytic interventions that this new theoretical perspective brings with it or at least somehow legitimates. To repeat an instance I heard about recently, which is admittedly rather extreme and that many relationalists themselves might condemn, a patient was telling her analyst a dream, and the analyst said to her patient, *"Your dream is giving me erotic feelings."* This was not an isolated incident in this analyst's practice: she seemed to revel in telling her patients such things, things which, to my way of thinking, reveal a tremendous amount about herself.

How, one might wonder, could such a statement be justified? Easily enough, it seems! It suffices to assume that if the analyst was feeling aroused, the patient was deliberately or unconsciously trying to turn her analyst on by talking about this particular dream. But what if the patient was just talking about this particular dream because she had just had it, and it seemed significant to her?

I don't know what it is like for those of you who are here in the audience today, but in my practice patients tell me all kinds of erotic dreams that do *not* turn me on, and others that do a bit now and then. Should I assume that my patients only intend to turn me on when their dreams actually turn me on and do not intend to turn me on when they don't? Isn't my being turned on or not when I hear someone's dream more a function of what turns me, Bruce Fink, on than my patient's conscious, preconscious, or unconscious intention to titillate me?

Many analysts from these newer traditions seem to enjoy being self-disclosing, and yet they somehow convince themselves that they are not *really* saying anything about themselves, since they believe that whatever they think or feel has been *put into them* by their analysands. Yet I suspect that most analysands would, when faced with an analyst who says, "Your dream is giving me erotic feelings," be convinced that such a remark says a good deal about the analyst! I suspect, too, that many analysands would feel creeped out or grossed out if their analyst made such a comment and decide to never talk about dreams like that again; other analysands, with a different psychology, might decide instead to talk about dreams like that on every possible occasion and in as much detail as possible! Both of these reactions would be quite unfortunate, skewing the analysis in potentially destructive ways.

Regarding self-disclosure (even when it is re-theorized as "objective countertransference" based on projective identification), let us recall that, as Lacan puts it, *all speech constitutes a demand for love*; so whenever we analysts speak, we are unconditionally asking to be heard (Seminar VIII, p. 356), we are asking for our words to be paid attention to—in short, we are asking to be loved.

This is one of the reasons why psychoanalysts must not speak too much during sessions, and must not reveal much about themselves, for when they do they are essentially asking or even begging, as Lacan (p. 370) puts it, to be loved; this is one of the many reasons why self-disclosure is such a bad idea. It is not so much in order to refuse to admit to be lacking that analysts must not speak so much, for analysis structurally puts analysts in the position of loving the analysand, and that loving itself reveals their lack. Analysis automatically places the analysand in the position of the beloved. The analysand, by speaking, demands to be found lovable, and we as analysts take the analysand as someone who is important and listen to him in a way that no one has ever listened to him before.

Analysts must not speak much in their own names or talk about themselves *so as not to demand to be loved in return by their analysands*. Freud himself was already aware of the danger involved in analysts wanting to be loved by their patients. He told Smiley Blanton (according to the latter's 1971 *Diary of my Analysis with Sigmund Freud*) that "Ferenczi tried to play the part of an overtender father, to give the love he himself had not received and to get love from his patients" (p. 67).[12]

You can perhaps guess where I am going with this: analysts, like everyone else, have failings, they all lack in some way. But analysts from these newer schools of psychoanalysis seem to be asking their patients to love them, not for the mountains of interpretations they have, as Freud did, but for their lack, for their flaws and failings—in a word, for their warts. It seems to me that by regularly bringing to the attention of patients the analysts' own feelings and sense of being pressured or cornered by the patient, analysts are asking to have their warts recognized by the patient, accepted by the patient, and indeed loved by the patient. In *Lacan on Love*, I wrote that "The analyst is far from taking expressions of the analysand's love for him at face value, does not seek out or relish the role of the beloved, and certainly does not wish to be loved for his 'subjective difference'" (2016, p. 51). I should have said that this is an ideal held primarily by Lacanian analysts, because I think it is pretty clear that analysts of a certain number of other persuasions have adopted a theory of practice that allows them to seek to be loved for their "subjective difference," that is, for their warts, in their own consulting rooms.

No one would, I think, dream of requiring analysts not to seek to be loved in their everyday lives, but many would, I think, ask analysts to forgo seeking love in the analytic setting. If we are seeking to be loved by our analysands for ourselves, we end up feeling that we exist only or primarily by being loved by them. This occasionally happens to therapists who allow themselves to be paged, called, or otherwise contacted by their patients day and night, spending much of their time returning their calls. It may seem that such therapists are reassuring their patients, or even mothering them, but the therapists are the ones who are being propped up and made to feel important. It is not just "Love and the Single Analyst" that can be problematic, as it is in the film *Sex and the Single Girl* (1964); married or not, in a "committed relationship" or not, practitioners who are unhappy or feel unloved outside of the consulting room are likely to begin looking for love in it.

In my informal surveys of analysands' views on the subject, they find it horrible or even disastrous when they sense that their analysts are wanting to be loved by them, such wanting often leading to the breaking off of the analysis.

This implies that the analyst's position is unique and paradoxical with respect to love, since, whereas love typically demands love in return, not being content to be unrequited, *the analyst must love without wanting to be loved in return*. Like Socrates, the analyst must refuse to adopt the position of the beloved in the analytic setting, striving instead to always be in the position of the lover.

MUTUAL MISSING
(MIS[T] SEXUAL RELATIONSHIP)

CHAPTER 5

Notions of love in Lacan's later work

(This material was presented at the end of a two-day workshop I gave on love, at the invitation of Eline Trenson, at the University of Ghent in Belgium on May 5–6, 2017.)

> *To become a psychoanalyst, one must be awfully taken with Freud, primarily—that is, one must believe in this absolutely crazy thing known as the unconscious, which I have tried to translate as the "subject-supposed-to-know."*
>
> —Lacan (1978b, p. 180)

In *Lacan on Love* (Fink, 2016), I only briefly discussed Lacan's views on love after the 1960s (see chapter 6). Yet Lacan broaches the topic of love at many different points and in many different contexts in the 1970s as well. For quite some time he attempts, as we shall see, to articulate what impact his oft-repeated conclusion that "there's no such thing as a sexual relationship" has on love. Does that mean, he wonders, that there's no such thing as love? Or that love somehow makes up for the missing sexual relationship? Lacan works this particular question over for several years.

Second, he remains intrigued by something he showed interest in at least as far back as Seminar VII, *The Ethics of Psychoanalysis*: the mystical tradition, and specifically the possible similarities and differences between what is known as *l'amour de Dieu*—divine love, which involves either God's love for us or our love for God, which is an "ecstatic" form of love—and other forms of love, whether love between couples or transference love. I will take this second topic up on another occasion.

I will make no attempt to be exhaustive in my discussion here and will refer you for that to Jean Allouch's excellent book entitled *L'amour Lacan* (2009), upon which I shall rely quite extensively. It cites virtually all of Lacan's discussions of love in the 1970s one by one, and attempts to put them together like pieces of a puzzle to create a theory of love that grows out of Lacan's work which is broader, at least in certain ways, than his earlier thesis of love as "giving what you don't have."

Neutrality versus smoldering

I will focus here especially on love as it manifests itself in the psychoanalytic context, and will begin by returning to a "myth" Lacan formulates in Seminar VIII regarding what he calls "the miracle of love" (discussed in chapter 3 of *Lacan on Love*). In Seminar VIII he concocts a "myth" about how love comes into being: love arises, he proposes, when we reach out toward an object—the examples he gives here being a flower, fruit, or log in a fire—and another hand reaches out toward us (pp. 51–52, 179). Presumably the miracle is that our love is reciprocated, the beloved reaching almost simultaneously for us. Lacan comments that "it is always inexplicable that anything whatsoever responds to [love]" (p. 52), which is why we need a myth. In other words, we cannot explain how the miracle of love occurs, how the beloved transforms into a lover; all we can do is provide an image for it.

Later in the same seminar, Lacan indicates that the hand that extends toward the log in the fire must do so with its own warmth or heat so that the flame leaps from the object, setting the object ablaze at its approach (pp. 388–389).[1] This warmth or heat is obviously the flame of desire: it is pure desirousness.

When it comes to the psychoanalytic setting, Lacan proposes that the analyst, who is not indifferent to the analysand's transference love, must not, however, burst into flames when the analysand expresses or manifests such love. The analyst is lucid about love, realizing that it involves the attempt to make one from two (*l'un d'eux, l'un deux*), to eradicate difference, something which is obviously impossible. Rather than bursting into flames, the analyst must find a way to *smolder*—that is, to burn without ever really catching on fire, like a log that is moist, if not completely soaked with rain. As he says,

> We all know that love's fires burn invisibly; we all know that a damp wooden beam can burn on the inside for a long time without anything being revealed on the outside. (p. 389)

If you have ever tried to build a fire with such wet wood, you are aware that it sizzles and pops, moisture turning to steam as it comes out of each end of the log, and that it is terribly difficult to get such moist logs to burst into flames. To the best of my knowledge, Lacan doesn't explicitly say that the analyst must merely smolder, but it is a possible extension of Lacan's notion. Allouch argues for it on the basis of Lacan's quip in 1960 in Brussels that he wanted to finish out his life by being "consumed" in the analytic armchair ("*À cette place, je souhaite qu'achève de se consumer ma vie*"); and on the basis of another comment he made in Italy regarding "*une consomption de mes jours*" ("a consuming of my days").[2] Unlike the burning bush which burned but was not consumed, the analyst is presumably consumed little by little, used up over time.[3]

Lacan did not endorse the notion of psychoanalytic "neutrality" as it was understood by his contemporaries. It might be argued that Freud introduced the notion that an analyst should manifest neutrality regarding any particular decision a patient makes, for example, to get married to a certain person or not. However, for many years in his consulting room, Freud was unable to stop himself from offering opinions about whom his patients should marry, and indeed offered opinions about a wide range of topics and decisions in his patients' lives, generally coming to regret having done so later. Indeed, in his "Papers on Technique" (SE XII), he formulated for the rest of us ordinary mortals the recommendation to keep our noses out of our patients' business in the sense of not proffering our own opinions about what they should do, and instead merely helping them articulate the pros and cons, and the unconscious desires and inhibitions at work in making such decisions.

The notion of neutrality was, however, taken up at times in the psychoanalytic community as a general affective or emotional attitude that should be adopted by analysts: one of indifference, of being unengaged, manifesting instead an almost robotic distance or coldness ("ataraxia," perfect tranquility or peace of mind, is the related term in Greek philosophy; Freud did say that "emotional coldness in the analyst" creates "for the doctor a desirable protection for his own emotional life" ["Recommendations to Physicians," SE XII, p. 115]; and mentions "the neutrality towards the patient, which we have acquired through keeping the counter-transference in check" ["Observations on Transference-Love," SE XII, p. 164]). Freud himself manifested anything but that in the analyses he conducted; in general, he was far too engaged with many of his patients, and not just the attractive hysterics he worked with, as I attempted to show in my *Clinical Introduction to Freud* (Fink, 2017; see, also, chapter 4 in the present collection).

Lacan, too, was, according to all accounts, anything but unengaged or coldly indifferent to his patients. In his theoretical work, Lacan countered the naïve and misguided notion, found in the French analytic literature of the time, of "well-meaning neutrality" (*neutralité bienveillante*), which is a formulation found nowhere in Freud's work,[4] with his own notion of *the analyst's desire*. That desire is not the personal desire of the analyst as a specific individual with his or her own quirks and characteristics, but rather a desire that is specifically related to the work of the analysis and that grows out of his or her fascination with the unconscious. It is a desire for analysands to come to their sessions, talk, dream, associate, and analyze—in short, to do the work of analysis. This is the kind of desire that can be expressed by analysts in which there is no ego anymore, as he expressed it early on (Seminar I, p. 287), by analysts who have given up their selves and gone through a form of mourning for themselves, analysts who can be characterized by a kind of *désêtre* (dis-being or un-being), instead of *être* (being), or who, at least in the analytic setting *put forward not their being but rather their lack of being*, not their own personality, but a generic desire for the analytic work to move forward.

Practitioners don't express such a desire as them*selves*, but as a function. If, as Lacan says, there is love only of a name (a bit of a curious claim on the face of it!), analysts don't name themselves, don't say who and what they are. Instead each analyst remains as opaque as possible throughout the analysis (Allouch, 2009, p. 450), not trying to be some special someone, but filling a generic role, a nameless, faceless role.[5]

This is a far cry from indifference, and I am surprised at times when patients who miss sessions or start talking about interrupting or stopping altogether their work with me seem to expect me to simply accept the breaking off of the analysis without any objection, thinking I couldn't care less whether they continue or not! While I am not indifferent, I am not personally invested in a big way in keeping the analysand close to me—that is, I am not personally invested in the way I hear about a great deal when I supervise analysts trained in other schools. Such analysts often feel personally thrilled when patients come to analysis, fall in love, and stay on, and personally hurt, abandoned, and/or criticized when they leave analysis. (What I try to do when they leave prematurely, in my view, is figure out what happened, why it happened just then, and keep that in mind in my future work.)

What is required on the analyst's part is to be neither indifferent nor personally involved, neither utterly ataraxic nor thrilled. The analyst must not fall in love with the analysand, even if the analyst *shows* love by listening to patients in a way that they have rarely if ever been listened to or paid attention to before, and remembering what they say in great detail over the course of many years. *What is required is that the analyst be in love with the unconscious*, that the analyst love the unconscious, as Lacan recommends we do in 1974 (Seminar XXI, class given on June 11, 1974), despite the pain in the neck (*emmerdements*) it gives us. The unconscious is, he says, a *"savoir emmerdant,"* an annoying knowledge, knowledge that is a pain in the ass.[6] The analyst must love the unconscious and seek to inspire love for the unconscious in his analysands.[7]

Many of the analysts I supervise seem confused about this, since their training does not emphasize getting at the unconscious but rather working everything out with the patient in the "here and now." They inevitably get enmeshed in rather messy erotic transferences and countertransferences with their patients. Rather than inspiring *a love for the unconscious* in their patients, they seem to inspire a love for themselves in their patients and become far too wrapped up in their patients' lives, decisions, struggles, and careers rather than in their patients' unconsciouses. This often leads to explosive situations and to the breaking off of treatment.

Lacan certainly doesn't say that analysts should have no feelings about their patients; he even goes so far as to say that it is not a very promising sign when analysts are never attracted to or angered by their patients. Analysts who have never felt the slightest temptation to have sex with their patients or harm them physically, he says in Seminar VIII, are perhaps not involved enough. As he puts it,

> I dare say that I wouldn't expect much from someone who has never felt [...] the desire to get down to it with his patient: to take him in his arms or throw him out the window. (Seminar VIII, p. 185)

But such feelings about their patients should be overridden by their desire as analysts to keep the work moving ahead.

> The analyst says, "I am possessed by a stronger desire." He is grounded in saying so as an analyst, insofar as a change has occurred in the economy of his desire. (Seminar VIII, p. 185)

In other words, the feelings analysts have for their patients—whether they temporarily take the form of love or hate, which are, as we know, but flip sides of each other—must merely smolder and not get the upper hand, not burst into flames and lead to an outburst of some kind. Love for the unconscious must take precedence over love for or hatred of the analysand.

We hope to inspire something similar in our patients. Although they may feel, especially at the outset, intrigued with us as their analysts (intrigued with who and what they think we are, which may turn to love and easily put an end to any real analytic work in the sessions), we attempt to convert that love for who they think we are into *love for what we stand in for, which is their own unconscious*. As Lacan puts it in his later work, *the subject-supposed-to-know is the unconscious—that is, the patient's unconscious* (Lacan, 1978b, p. 180). Through our own focus on the unconscious during sessions, we endeavor to incite in them a love, not for ourselves as living breathing human beings with our own peculiarities and foibles, but rather for their own unconscious. We agree to stand in for the unknown knowledge within themselves, which they project onto us as if we knew it in advance, whereas all we know is how to try to bring it out. Insofar as they love the subject-supposed-to-know, they come to love their own unconscious.

What is it like to love someone—an analyst—who loves the unconscious, despite all the trouble it brings with it? Is that what we love him for, or are we frustrated that he loves something other than what we think of as ourselves? Love in the analytic setting is *limited* by the fact that analysts *love something other than us* (and not just their spouses, children, pets, or other patients; Allouch, 2009, p. 405). To love, in the analytic setting, is to love two very different things: the analyst and the unconscious, or (in the case of the analyst) the analysand and the unconscious. Love for the unconscious keeps love for the other party to the analytic adventure moderate, not excessive.[8]

Getting something without really getting it

This connects up with another component of Lacan's later work on love, which is that in analysis one obtains love without really obtaining it (Allouch, 2009, p. 436). If one *really* obtains it, in other words, if one somehow manages to actually seduce the analyst and receive his or her love, whether it is manifested physically or otherwise, then the analysis has failed.

A great many people come to analysis feeling that they have never been sufficiently recognized or loved by their family, friends, teachers, or bosses, and hope to win such recognition or love from their analyst. Although we analysts, in paying very close attention to what they tell us, recognize them as people worth listening to, we are best advised to *not* give them signs of love that go beyond the analytic work itself. Thus they often feel that they have not gotten the kind of unconditional parental love they were hoping for, proofs of which they are often seeking in any little thing we do that might seem a little bit out of the ordinary, to go just a tad beyond the frame that we appear to have set for the analytic work, wishing to see in it a proof that we love them more than we are willing to say. For some, this goes so far as to fantasize that we want them sexually and are coming on to them, subtly or not so subtly, because in their lives that was the way people around them showed them special favor.

Although we do not give them the kind or quantity of love they are seeking, in the best of cases we arouse in them love for the unconscious. They do not get the love that they think they want from us, which, were they to get it, would probably scare them, be overwhelming, and almost certainly put an end to the analysis, but we incite in them love for something else, for the unconscious. We seek to make it possible for them to love someone outside of the analytic setting, that is, someone other than ourselves (as Socrates says to Alcibiades: love Agathon, not me!), but we also seek to inspire in them a love for the unconscious.

In this way, they obtain something which at the same time they do not exactly obtain; they get something without actually getting it. They want to be loved but end up loving. Is it a game of bait and switch?

The same is true when it comes to knowledge. Patients sometimes claim at the outset of their analyses that they want to figure out why such and such happened in their lives and why they do certain things that they cannot fathom—for example, why they repeat the same patterns over and over again. In the course of their analyses, we help them develop all kinds of associations and speculations in response to their questions, but we rarely if ever are able to bring them to the point of feeling they have some kind of absolute knowledge about why they did what they did and became what they became. Their quest for absolutely certain knowledge is thwarted or disappointed, and yet, in the best of cases, they come away with knowledge that seems adequate to them, knowledge that is *good enough* for their purposes, realizing that the other kind is either simply a pipe dream or no longer of any interest to them. They come away with a sort of *docta ignorantia*, learned ignorance (as in *educated* ignorance).

Freud wanted, in the case of his patient Elfriede Hirschfeld (but probably in other cases as well), to reveal to her what he believed to be the ultimate or final truth, the absolute truth about her illness, its most secret *raison d'être*, but she broke off her analysis instead (Falzeder, 1994, p. 309)![9] Lacan calls this *"la connerie de la vérité,"* "the idiocy of truth." A piece of knowledge cannot be put in the place of truth, cannot serve as some sort of absolute truth—there can only be partial truths and bits of knowledge. Lacan was quite aware that Freud's approach to interpretation was often misguided, aiming as it did, especially early on in his work, at simply conveying a piece or chunk of supposed knowledge or truth to patients, without taking the time to bring them to formulate it themselves. And what analysands themselves formulate remains open to question and qualification indefinitely; it never becomes absolute, yet, with luck, they come to no longer care whether it is absolute or not.

In this sense, patients obtain knowledge in the course of their analyses, without really obtaining it; they get what they came for without getting exactly what they came for. This is part of what Lacan (1981) calls *"l'escroquerie psychanalytique,"* the analytic con game or rip off. As we see in the case of Elfriede Hirschfeld, if you actually get what you thought you came for (or sense that you are about to get it), you run the other way. Lacan says repeatedly that our stance as human beings is essentially, "Don't give me what I ask for because that's not it, it's not really what I want!" (Freud tried to give Hirschfeld what he thought he had, an S_2, knowledge, instead of what he didn't have.) This mustn't be taken to mean that Lacan thinks we should never interpret. For he says that,

> It is insofar as an apt interpretation puts an end to [or: resolves, *éteint*] a symptom that truth shows itself to be poetic [or: proves to be poetic]. (Seminar XXIV, class given on April 19, 1977)

Lacan thus continues to tout the importance of interpretation right up until the end of his teaching, as well as the possibility of symptom resolution. But such "apt" interpretations usually don't set out to deliver an S_2 as such, a precise piece of knowledge. Their aim is, instead, to make waves, to have an impact.[10]

Love is getting what hasn't been given

We can begin to see here how this might link up with Lacan's earlier formulation of love as "giving what you don't have." If to love is to give what you don't have, the beloved receives something that has not exactly been given. The beloved somehow gets something that hasn't been handed over, whether that be knowledge or "proofs" of love. The analyst does not hand over knowledge and yet the analysand comes away knowing something of great importance. The analyst does not give love or recognition directly and yet the analysand may well come away loving his or her unconscious and feeling like someone pretty special.

L'amour fou, *crazy love*

> *Le "faire deux" des amants est ce qui les met "hors d'eux."*
> If lovers can't become one, remaining two instead, they get furious!
> —Lacan, Seminar XXI, class given on December 18, 1973

This approach to love in psychoanalysis offers up quite a different picture of love than the one Lacan believes has prevailed for millennia: *l'amour fou*, crazy or passionate love, a kind of love that has been celebrated since at least ancient Greek times. This is the kind we see in Aristophanes' myth of beings who, after having been split into two by

Zeus, find their other halves and meld with each other, melt into each other, unify. What this crazy or passionate kind of love seeks to accomplish, according to Lacan, is *de deux faire un*, to make two into one. On the basis of two thoroughly separate individuals, it seeks to make but one, and a one that is not missing anything, a one that is whole, lacking in nothing, uncastrated. This notion is connected to Freud's notion of narcissistic love in which one loves another as part of oneself or loves oneself in another. Crazy or passionate love seeks to bring about a feeling of fusion between lovers, and generally fails to do so for more than short periods of time.

When it does bring about a more enduring sense of fusion, we are usually dealing with psychosis. Recall that in psychosis, we find a specific configuration when it comes to belief. Whereas neurotics tend to believe what other people say only within certain limits, and even tend to believe what they themselves say only within certain limits (doubt and self-doubt being major hallmarks of neurosis), psychotics tend to believe certain things utterly and completely, believing certain people in a wholehearted way and believing what they themselves say in a similarly total way.

Lacan finds a parallel here with the phenomenon of "crazy love" even in people who are not psychotic. He mentions men and women who fall in love with a woman who becomes both a sort of God and a symptom for them, qualifying this phenomenon with the curious abbreviation FOS, for *femme ondine symptôme*, a woman as an undine (a sort of mythological water spirit, nymph, or goddess) and a symptom. He makes a distinction here between *y croire*—believing in her, for example, believing such a goddess exists—and *la croire*, believing everything she says. In crazy love, people begin to believe everything such a woman says.[11]

This is where crazy love and the analyst's love part company: the analyst believes in the patient, believes that the patient is trying to tell him or her something in his or her own peculiar way, but always remains at one remove from the story, always remembering that there is probably more to the story than is being told, and that the story may in fact be completely false. If the patient claims to hear voices, the analyst believes that the patient hears the voices, but does not believe what the voices say.

In loving the analysand, the analyst does not go as far as people do in crazy love: he or she never goes so far as to believe everything the analysand says, or even to completely believe virtually *anything* the analysand says, always maintaining a certain modicum of skepticism or disbelief. Here again, love in the analytic setting is not that of crazy fusion, but something else (Seminar XXII, class given on January 21, 1975, and Allouch, 2009, pp. 360–364).

Nor does the patient believe whatever the analyst says, at least in most cases. And the analyst certainly does not ask him or her to! If the analyst professes to know everything, then there is no room for the subject-supposed-to-know, which is only maintained by *not* dispensing knowledge, not interpreting everything (Allouch, 2009, pp. 362–363).

Although one would think that Lacan had sufficiently critiqued crazy love (an imaginary form of love based on narcissism) by the mid- to late 1950s, with his formulation of a more symbolic form of love as giving what you don't have—that is, as giving something related to lack and symbolic castration—in the 1970s he keeps coming back to this fusional form of love, to the idea of two becoming one. This concern with the one of fusion can be seen in his often repeated claim in the 1970s, "*Il y a de l'Un*," "there is such a thing as One," One here typically being capitalized. This is usually understood at the level of signifiers, there being such a thing as the signifier one or S_1,[12] but Lacan also enjoins the analyst not to take him- or herself as a one, as some one (*être quelqu'un*), as a specific, special individual in the analyses he or she conducts, but rather as playing something of a generic role (unspecified as this one or that one), the role of object *a*.

Note too that *être quelqu'un* in French means to be someone who is very important, to be a big macher, a big kahuna, which is precisely what analysts must not think they are, at least while they are practicing psychoanalysis. Thinking of themselves as people who are terribly important clearly gets in the way of allowing themselves to become scraps that are sloughed off or left by the wayside by the analysand in the course of the analysis (i.e., to undergo subjective destitution or *désêtre*). The more analysts put them*selves* forward, the less they stand in for their patients' unconscious.

Love and the nonexistence of a sexual relationship

> Psychoanalysis … is a bond between two people [*lien à deux*]. That is why it is found in the place of the missing sexual relationship.
>
> —Lacan, 1975d, p. 187

I mentioned earlier that Lacan's bombshell declaration, first made on March 12, 1969, toward the end of Seminar XVI, that "there's no such thing as a sexual relationship," no logically definable relationship between the sexes, had quite an impact on his own theory, not just on his audience. He presents this as the very thing that patients complain about endlessly on the couch: that no matter how hard they try, they cannot actually establish any sort of meaningful connection or relationship with their partner of the opposite sex insofar as that partner is of the opposite sex. They can have sex; they can be friends; they can act like siblings toward each other; and they can interact with each other as though they were parent and child; but they cannot establish a relationship with each other based on sexual difference or sexuation. In other words, there is such a thing as a relationship between friends, between siblings, and between parents and children, but there is no such thing as a relationship between the sexes insofar as they are men and women.

Where does that leave love? There is such a thing as what the Greeks called *philia*, love between friends, which Aristotle defines as wishing the other well and wanting what is best for the other; there is such a thing as brotherly or sisterly love; there is such a thing as parental and filial love; and there may even be love for one's neighbor, known as Christian love; but what about love between partners? Obviously there is *some* kind of love between partners, but does it have any connection with their sex?

Certain trends in modern culture attempt to decree that love and sex *must* go hand in hand, that the person with whom we have sexual enjoyment must also be the person we love. We even have a tendency to believe (perhaps less so today, however) that we cannot experience sexual enjoyment with someone unless we love that person. Lacan disagrees with this, saying, in the very first class of Seminar XX, that "enjoyment of the body of the other person who symbolizes the Other for us [*la jouissance de l'Autre*], is not the sign of love" (p. 4). Sexually enjoying another person's body is not a sign—much less *the* sign—of our love for that person. Such enjoyment can exist without love, and love can exist without such enjoyment.

Lacan tries out a number of different ways of formulating the connection between love and the nonexistence of the sexual relationship, several of them in Seminar XX alone.

On January 16, 1973, he suggests that love is the signified of the signifier "sexual relationship." In the same class he also proposes that love makes up for, or compensates us for the absence of the sexual relationship. We are distressed by our inability to establish any such relationship, and love provides us with a kind of supplement or compensation.

On June 26, 1973, at the end of Seminar XX, he proposes that love appears *because* of our confrontation with the absence of the sexual relationship. It supposedly suspends the sexual relationship and allows for recognition of the partner in a subject-to-subject relationship. The idea here is that the male-to-female connection is set aside or overwritten in favor of a relationship between two beings that has nothing to do with their respective sexes. Sexual difference is rendered irrelevant when love comes into the picture; the absence of a sexual relationship is ignored by the partners to such a subject-to-subject relationship, whether they are heterosexual, homosexual, bi, or whatever. The subject-to-subject relationship seems to overcome love as *l'(a)mur*, which was how Lacan wrote love for quite some time, believing there to be a kind of wall (*mur*) between lovers, a wall somehow related to object *a*. Instead of a wall, this subject-to-subject relationship seems to be something that links lovers to each other, but *not* insofar as they are sexed beings.

Lacan refers to this as a new sort of love (1975a, p. 16; see, also, Soler, 2003), which involves recognition of the way in which the partner is affected by his or her unconscious, a love that takes into account the partner's unconscious instead of trying not to see it, as people generally do. It promises a relationship between two unconscious knowledges, so to speak: a relationship between the knowledge situated in my unconscious and the knowledge situated in my partner's unconscious, as if we somehow recognized each other's unconsciouses via a certain set of signs related to symptoms—symptoms of our partner's "exile from the sexual relationship," which is true of us too.[13] To be willing to recognize those signs is thus to love. (There are plenty of families that seem to willfully overlook or ignore obvious symptoms in certain family members—not a very loving attitude, to say the least.)

There seems to be something rather optimistic here for once as regards love (even if Allouch [2009, p. 348] considers it to be a mirage). Lacan goes so far as to hint, perhaps, that his patients notice signs of *his* unconscious, in the guise of his *"je n'en veux rien savoir"* ("I don't want to know anything about it"; Seminar XX, p. 1), which they perceive to be different from their own. We might then consider transference love to be based on signs that analysands perceive of their analyst's unconscious, and indeed certain analysands fixate on any little slip or slurring of words they believe their analyst makes or the slightest bungling of things on the analyst's part, in an attempt to guess at what it might be a sign of (usually as concerns themselves, however).

Lacan almost never returns to the idea of a subject-to-subject relationship, except to say, a couple of months later:

> It is entirely conceivable that you may have, with someone you love, some unconscious relations. But it is not insofar as you love that person that you have such relations, because insofar as you love that person, *on la râte*, you miss him or her, you don't reach [or: hit or attain, *atteindre*] him or her. (Seminar XXI, class given on November 2, 1973)

In other words, when Lacan does come back to the idea of a subject-to-subject relationship, he dissociates it from love, strictly speaking; perhaps what he means there is that it has absolutely nothing to do with libido, which always somehow misses its object. To Lacan's way of thinking, love (as eros or libido) has to do with *missing*, failure, or messing up, and seems here to get in the way of recognizing the unconscious of one's partner. The subject-to-subject relationship perhaps has something to do, instead, for Lacan, with *philia* or Christian love.[14]

A few weeks later, he adds:

> Love is two half-sayings that do not intersect [or: overlap]. This is what makes them lethal (*fatales*). We have here an irremediable division […], a connection between two knowledges [i.e., two different people's knowledge] insofar as they are irremediably distinct. (Seminar XXI, class given on January 15, 1974)

The modal articulation of love and the nonexistence of the sexual relationship

In Seminar XX, Lacan also tries to base the relationship between love and the nonexistence of the sexual relationship on modal logic (involving possibility, impossibility, necessity, and contingency), which he had recently become fascinated with, coming up with a highly complex model that looks more or less like this:

A) The sexual relationship *ne cesse pas de ne pas s'écrire* (never stops not being written). This means that sexual relationships are *impossible*.
B) The "illusion" brought on by love is that the sexual relationship *cesse de ne pas s'écrire* (stops not being written). When one stops dwelling on the impossibility of such a relationship, love can appear; it doesn't *have* to appear, but it may appear. If one happens upon the right person, if a certain *contingent* encounter occurs, love may come into the picture, but what it involves is a subject-to-subject relationship.
C) Love *ne cesse pas de s'écrire* (never stops being written): we see here the poetic striving to make love last forever, seem necessary, and not contingent. It is not that we just happened to meet by accident: it was fated to be, we were made for each other, it was written in the stars!
D) The category of the possible is less developed in this context. It would seem to imply that the sexual relationship (or, perhaps, love) *cesse de s'écrire* (stops being written).

It is, Allouch (2009, p. 358) suggests, the very nonexistence of the sexual relationship that makes love necessary. Is this sublimation in Freud's sense? You don't have satisfying sex so you have to love?

Let us note that in Seminar XXII (class given on February 11, 1975), Lacan concludes that love and the sexual relationship have absolutely nothing to do with each other![15]

SOMETHING IS *a*-MISS

CHAPTER 6

Why people aren't what they seem to be, or what Freud teaches us about repression

(This talk was given, at the invitation of Stephanie Swales, to an audience of mostly undergraduates at the University of Dallas on November 2, 2018.)

Why do the very people who initially seem to be the most laid-back and mild-mannered sometimes turn out to be hateful monsters who end up stabbing you in the back? Why is it that someone you thought was totally and devotedly in love with you fails to show up at the date you had, completely forgets to do the favor he said he would do for you, or suddenly betrays you without you having seen it coming?

Are most people consummate actors who know full well that they are duping you? Some of them undoubtedly are, but Freud suggests that many of them may in fact be duping themselves. And he teaches us plenty of ways to see how and when they are doing so.

I will begin with a number of familiar facts, some of which psychologists were aware of long before Freud's time, and others that Freud himself uncovered and tried to account for.

Common occurrences

1) Your partner accuses you of cheating on him or at least of flirting with others and wanting to cheat on him. You, on the other hand, are incredibly in love with him and haven't thought about anyone else in weeks, if not months. What often turns out to be the case is that *it is your partner* who has been dreaming and/or daydreaming about other people. He is perhaps not even consciously aware he has been doing so, and can only think about cheating insofar as he attributes the impulse to you. Or perhaps he is aware he has been doing so, and is angry at himself, but gets angry at you instead. Something that he refuses to see or reckon with in himself is attributed by him to you, he not wanting to take responsibility for it. Freud considered this to be a typical example of what he called "projection," and noted that those who manifest the most jealousy are often those who have the most uncontrollably roving eyes.

2) You are a very good driver and yet every time you are about to leave home your mother goes on and on about how careful you should be on the road and how worried she is every time you get in a car. Why is she constantly thinking about you getting into a wreck? Have you given her any reason to worry you will have an accident? Or did she herself once get into a bad wreck? If not, she may be constantly imagining that for her own reasons … Now what might those be? Maybe she would secretly like something bad to happen to you, because then you might need her to take care of you like you did when you were little and she is missing that. Perhaps you drive her crazy and so something in her would like to see something bad happen to you. Maybe her feelings for you are not as lovey-dovey as she would like to convince you they are!

   Aggressive thoughts that people have about each other are very often expressed out loud as worries or anxieties. I have heard many patients tell me they are worried their fathers will have a heart attack, and when I ask whether their fathers have been ill lately or whether there is any history of heart disease in the family, they say no. In fact, they have no reason whatsoever to think their fathers will have a heart attack, and yet they often "worry" about that, being "anxious" about their fathers' health. Freud suggests that *anger* at or *resentment* of their fathers has, in such cases, been transformed into worry or anxiety, which serves as a disguise. Indeed, Freud goes so far as to suggest that all of the emotions we have that we refuse to acknowledge and for which we do not wish to accept responsibility may well be transformed in us into anxiety, anxiety being what he calls "the universal currency" of all affect ("the universally current coinage," SE XVI, pp. 403–404; "affect" is Freud's main term for emotion or feeling). Every feeling that we push out of mind, whether love or hate, attraction or fear, can be converted into anxiety. Indeed, when you ask people why they are anxious or what they are anxious about, they often have no clue; or if they think they have a clue, it is often a side issue or a "false connection" (SE II, p. 67 n.) that has little or nothing to do with the real source of their anxiety.

3) Someone I know is a very straight-laced, no-nonsense, retired high school teacher who tends to dress like the stereotypical librarian. One day she was invited to a wedding party, got rip-roaring drunk, jumped up on the table, and began dancing like a banshee! Not even her husband had ever seen her like that before. When inhibitions are lifted, another side of people often shows itself. People have a tendency to suppress a lot of things that they feel and would like to do, but when they drink enough or take enough drugs, the impulses they have been pushing out of sight or suppressing tend to get the upper hand.

Which one is the real you? The one who suppresses everything you feel or the one who goes nuts, drinks like a freshman on spring break, and dances on tables?

4) Your girlfriend fails to show up at the library where you were supposed to meet and when you ask her about it, she goes into so much detail about the supposed event that made it impossible for her to show up that you begin to wonder if it isn't in fact an elaborate deception. If it were true that she had been asked to drive a pregnant woman to the emergency room, why would she be saying so much about it, repeating herself and, in essence, saying way more than she needs to about it, excessively justifying herself? In the attempt to pull the wool over your eyes, she invents a million minute details, whereas she could have simply told you that she'd been asked to drive someone to the ER and could have counted on you to believe her. Instead she was probably doing something she either wasn't terribly proud of or thinks you would heartily disapprove of. The more she embellishes the story, the more she arouses your suspicions.

5) Your boyfriend tells you, "I really really really really really love you," repeating the term "really" so many times that your ears perk up. After all, when people overemphasize their feelings in this way, we know from experience that the word "but" is rarely far behind: "I really really really really really love you, but you drive me crazy," "but I met someone else," etc.

6) Your supposed girlfriend tells you, "That outfit you're wearing is *so* fab!" when she finds it horrendous or laughable, and then turns around and makes a vomiting gesture you can't see to another friend behind her so that the latter will realize she doesn't believe a word of it. We try to deceive other people by saying the exact opposite of what we really think or feel, but we tend to give that away by the very excessive nature of our comment. "Oh, I just *loved* your class presentation!" often means "What a snore!" "That birthday present you bought me was *so* thoughtful" often means "I regifted it as soon as I could."

7) Your teacher says, "I don't mean to be critical," and virtually everyone knows from experience that such a comment is bound to be followed by the word "but" and a severe criticism. "I don't mean to be rude, but" is usually followed by an incredibly rude remark or gesture. People seem to think that by denying that they have a certain intention, their remarks won't be taken as critical or rude, but few people are duped by this. Freud was probably the first to say that the best way to understand such "unprovoked denials" (see Fink, 2007, pp. 41–42) is to simply cross out the word "not" in them:

"I do ~~not~~ mean to be critical" = "I mean to be quite critical."

8) You think you hate someone, and don't realize that you perhaps also love them until you have a dream in which you find yourself passionately kissing them. You wake up thinking that was bizarre and gross, but perhaps little by little you begin to wonder if it perhaps meant something (patients frequently tell me such dreams). Love and hate are often intimately related, one being the flip side of the other.

9) You have a professor who seems to be one of the most laid back and relaxed people you have ever met. You take all of his classes and for years you even go to the meditation groups he organizes every week.

You decide to do your master's thesis with him, you go over all of the material and reading lists with him, and agree on how to approach things in the thesis. You write the paper, hand it in, and lo and behold, he gives you a bad grade—indeed, a grade so low that even if the two other readers of the thesis gave you an A, you would still fail. Your professor seemed to be so easygoing and to love absolutely everything you did, but he turned around and screwed you over royally. Which one of those was the real him: the Dalai Lama or the backstabber?

Perhaps his laid-back demeanor was nothing more than a put on, but perhaps he had convinced himself that he was a peace-loving, easygoing guy who had reached such a state of spiritual perfection that he had verily and truly eliminated all aggression within himself. We should be suspicious of such displays of perfection—for perfection rarely if ever exists in reality—and the more someone tries to portray himself as serene and unperturbable, the more he is likely to be a cauldron of boiling passions underneath. Maybe the professor had fallen in love with you and punished you for the fact that he couldn't allow himself to be with you without losing his job; maybe he punished you because his attraction to you created a great deal of tension with his partner; or maybe he punished you because he had such high hopes for your master's thesis that you couldn't possibly have lived up to his ridiculously overblown expectations, he having wanted you to write the book he should have written but never got around to writing. (This recently happened to a friend of mine.)

Opposites attract

Freud concluded from many such occurrences that, in human beings, opposites are very closely related to each other: that it is the person you love the most passionately that you end up hating the most fervently, and that the person you profess to hate the most loudly is the one you may end up hooking up with; that when someone screams, "You're cheating on me," it often means "I'm cheating on you"; that when people want someone dead or to get hurt, they sometimes express worry about his health instead, or express a need to protect that person—from whom we might ask? From themselves!

Indeed, Freud went so far as to propose that the conscious and the unconscious are generally the exact opposite of each other: "the unconscious is the precise contrary of the conscious," he wrote (SE X, p. 180).

When a patient says, "My younger sister didn't mean anything to me growing up," it is often far truer that "she meant the world to me." When he says, "My brother was of no importance to me growing up," as one of my patients did in an early session with me, it often turns out that his brother was the bane of his existence, beat him up, tortured him, and had a huge influence on the direction his life took. We may represent such situations as follows, where what is under the bar (or fraction-like line) is unconscious and what is above it is conscious:

$$\frac{\text{"I hate you"}}{\text{I love you}}$$

$$\frac{\text{"You're cheating on me"}}{\text{You're loyal to me but }I'm\text{ cheating on you}}$$

$$\frac{\text{"I'm worried about your health"}}{\text{I hope you croak; I want you out of my life}}$$

$$\frac{\text{"My sister meant nothing to me"}}{\text{My sister meant everything to me}}$$

$$\frac{\text{"My brother was of no importance to me growing up"}}{\text{My brother was the bane of my existence}}$$

Freud concluded from such examples that:

> Opposite thoughts are always closely connected with each other and are often paired in such a way that *the one thought* [e.g., "I'm worried about your health"] *is excessively, intensely conscious while its opposite is repressed and unconscious.* (SE VII, p. 55)

Theoretical discussion of the conscious and unconscious

We can think about the relation between what is conscious and what is unconscious in a number of different ways.

Jacques Lacan proposed that we can, in a sense, view conscious and unconscious as like two sides of a Möbius strip, on opposite sides from each other locally, but if we follow one far enough, we arrive at the other (see Figure 6.1).

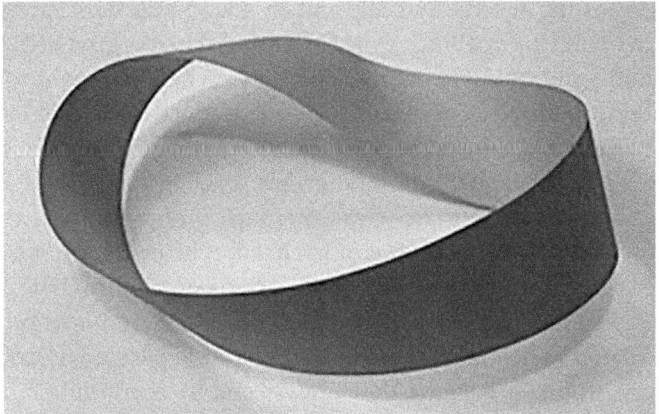

Figure 6.1: A Möbius strip

Freud, for his part, often thought of the unconscious as a kind of depth, something deep down and dark, and used the metaphor of an archeological dig to talk about it, the idea being that analyst and analysand slowly delve into the depths of the psyche and dust off this bit of the unconscious and then that bit, going ever deeper.

But Freud also showed how close the unconscious can at times be to the surface, so to speak, as when someone makes a slip of the tongue. Slips of the tongue can at times be simply confusing and opaque, as for example when one means to say, "I could really go for a hamburger now," and instead says, "I could really go for a jamburger now." The person who made the slip might be able to tell us that she had been thinking about a jam session she had been to, or a new type of jelly she had tried, or a guy named Joe or Jamie, but most people listening to her will have no idea what her slip reveals.

Yet, if the same person is thanking you for having helped her out of a difficult situation and she suddenly slips and says, "I could just kill you," when the context seemed to indicate that she was about to say, "I could just kiss you," almost everybody will be a bit taken aback and wonder what the heck just happened. Freud would suggest that she perhaps unconsciously harbors some resentment against you, perhaps because she was annoyed that she wasn't able to get out of the difficult situation herself and needed your help, but perhaps for other reasons as well, and that her resentment was able to slip out owing in part to the similarity of the two words "kiss" and "kill."

Sometimes the words that slip out in such "mistakes" aren't very similar in sound or spelling, as for example when a guy says that he was "talking with a hot brunette" at a party when he meant to say he was "talking with a hot redhead." Freud proposes that there is probably some brunette who was on his mind—perhaps not consciously—whether it was his sister, his mother, his teacher, or his best friend's girlfriend, a brunette who he would perhaps prefer not to be thinking about but whom he can't get out of his head. A brunette is not the exact opposite of a redhead, in the way that we think of love and hate as exact opposites, but they were perhaps closely associated in his mind nevertheless, insofar as he may have been trying for the past few years to stay away from brunettes because they always end up reminding him of his mother and his sister.

Freud suggested that at times we can pretty easily figure out what other people are really thinking by paying close attention to the slips of the tongue they make (e.g., the president of a club who was supposed to say, "I officially declare this meeting open" instead said he officially declared it "closed" even before it started, as if he wanted it to be over with already; SE XV, p. 34), as well as the slip-ups they make in everyday life, like "forgetting" about a date they have with you, showing up on your doorstep on the wrong day, accidentally leaving their diary in your apartment, and so on.

Freud mentions a striking slip-up in his *Introductory Lectures on Psychoanalysis*: a famous German chemist decides to get married; one day he gets dressed for work, goes to his lab, and spends all day working on his experiments. Only later does he realize that it was his wedding day and that his wife-to-be and her friends and family were expecting him at church! He concludes that he didn't really want to get married anyway, and you can imagine that his fiancée probably concluded the same thing (SE XV, p. 58). Freud calls such slip-ups "bungled actions" or "parapraxes," and one can hardly imagine a more telling one.

Someone who has a guilty conscience may "accidentally" leave proof of his infidelity behind, "forgetting" his phone in your room, perhaps secretly hoping to be found out. He may assume that you won't be able to resist the temptation to look through his texts and phone messages, and then the cat will be out of the bag. He may deny until he's blue in the face that he had any such intention, but then why did he leave his phone behind on that particular occasion, whereas he never goes anywhere without it? Freud concludes that there are no "accidents": what was not consciously intended was unconsciously intended. Maybe he wanted to end things with you, or maybe he just wanted to get his infidelity out in the open and see if you would force him to put an end to it. Maybe it was a test to find out how much he means to you: would you stick it out with him and try to make things work again between you?

People sometimes deliberately leave a book or purse behind in someone's home so that they'll have an excuse to go back there. In the case of the unfaithful boyfriend who leaves his phone behind in your room, it probably isn't consciously deliberate and yet it is perhaps motivated by something like a guilty conscience and an unconscious wish or a faintly perceived wish to come clean or to bring on a break-up.

If the unfaithful boyfriend who leaves behind his phone in your room were to lie on the couch and talk openly with a psychoanalyst, he might admit to having been uncomfortable with the situation as it was, couldn't think of a way to talk with his girlfriend about what was going on, and yet wanted some resolution. We need not think of all of the contents of the unconscious as so deeply buried that it takes years to uncover any one of them. Sometimes, when certain surprising or counterintuitive thoughts come out in the course of someone's analysis, the person comments that he has always been dimly aware of that, always sort of knew it, but never really allowed himself to face it until he said it out loud in a session. He was vaguely aware of it but put it out of mind. A female analysand of mine recently admitted—after having a dream in which she had horrible blisters all over her legs—that there are things about herself that she considers terribly ugly but diligently hides from everyone. It takes a lot of energy to hide certain things and sometimes we might like to simply throw off the mask and let the chips fall where they may! It's as if she were thinking, "Let's see who will still like me if I show my true colors."

Putting something out of mind

What exactly does it mean to put something out of mind? Let's say you have an exam in three hours and you get some disturbing news about someone in your family. You attempt to put it out of mind with the idea that you'll deal with it after the exam. It may still plague you a bit while you're trying to cram for the exam and even while you are taking the exam; you are obviously still conscious of it and will turn your attention to it as soon as the exam is over. Yet human beings are able to put things out of mind in a much more encompassing and enduring way as well. They are able to do so in ways that make the thing being put out of mind more or less unavailable and inaccessible—at least without hypnosis in certain cases, and without psychoanalysis in many cases.

The result of putting things out of mind in this more encompassing and perhaps even permanent way is very often the formation of a symptom. If I am extremely angry with a parent who criticizes me all the time and threatens me with slaps and punches, and who nevertheless is the only parent I've got, I may well squelch my desire to strike back at my parent. Instead, I may hide my anger to the point that the only visible sign of it that remains is a nervous tic. What form do such tics usually take? My eyes blink, my teeth clench, a muscle in my jaw twitches, or my head makes jerky movements whenever I am reminded in any way of my anger at this parent. Few people seem to pay attention to this, but many of the nervous tics that children develop sketch out the very beginning of ducking motions, as if they were about to dodge a blow coming from someone, or prepare for a blow from someone by closing their eyes, thereby protecting them; or, in a different vein, that sketch out hitting or biting motions, as if they wanted to hit or bite but then suppress that urge.

We see here an urge to strike out at someone which is combated by a counter urge. The urge to attack one's parent is suppressed, and the war between these two urges gives rise to something that is generally unrecognizable either to the parent or to the child: a "compromise formation," as Freud called it. Everyone around the child is aware that something is amiss, that something has gone awry, but most people are incapable of saying what it is.

$$\text{Urge 1} \Rightarrow \text{symptom} \Leftarrow \text{Urge 2}$$

$$\text{Force 1} \Rightarrow \text{symptom} \Leftarrow \text{Force 2}$$

Freud gave an example of a young woman who was devotedly taking care of her father who had fallen ill. His illness lasted quite a long time, got worse and worse, and she tended to him day and night for months on end. One day she heard music with a fine dance beat coming from the house next door, and it made her think she'd rather be out dancing with some young neighbors than staying up all night watching over her father. But this thought seemed utterly reprehensible to her—how could she possibly wish for such a thing when her father was in such a bad way? She did her best to suppress this wish, and curiously enough began coughing whenever she heard music with a good beat. The coughing covered over the music—in other words, she could barely hear the music anymore due to her own coughing, as if she were hoping to forget she had ever heard music that sparked a wish in her to do something other than care for her father. The coughing persisted until she was finally able to say when it first started and under what conditions. Speaking that out loud to her doctor put an end to the coughing symptom (SE II, pp. 43–44).

We can hypothesize here that when her nervous cough developed, her wish to go out dancing (Wish 1, or W_1 for short) was repressed, isolated, or cut off from conscious awareness. In particular, it was cut off from her conscious wish to be a model daughter and take perfect care of her father (Wish 2, or W_2):

$$W_1 \mid W_2$$

Stuttering can be the result of much the same process of having a wish or an impulse and squelching it: wanting to yell at or insult someone and suppressing that impulse.[1]

Humans have at their disposal a mechanism so strong that it can put both impulses—the impulse to strike out at someone and the counter-impulse or squelching impulse—out of mind quite completely, so strong that it can lead to the formation of symptoms that last a lifetime. Common examples of these are the fear of flying,[2] the fear of elevators and other small spaces, the fear of dogs, the fear of spiders, the fear of heights, the fear of open spaces, the fear of crossing bridges over water, etc. These fears or phobias are differently motivated in different cases, but they very often involve a fear of being swallowed up or devoured by one of one's parents.[3] And once they form, they have a tendency to last throughout one's entire adult life, without the person who has the fear or phobia having much of an idea at all why it formed and what the warring forces involved in it are. If, after all, they were aware of W_2—their wish to squelch W_1—then they'd know something about W_1, and they don't want to know anything about that! So, they have to forget both, W_1 and W_2.

Freud termed this incredibly strong mechanism "repression." Repression remains a hypothetical notion to this day, as the exact nature of repression remains to be fleshed out. What does it mean to put something out of mind so thoroughly that it is completely forgotten and inaccessible? And what does it take for something that has been put out of mind in this way, that is, that has been repressed, to come back to mind?

Trying too hard

Let's begin with a simple example of repression, one that involves "trying too hard," and in which it was not that difficult to bring back to mind what had been put out of mind.

One of my patients, who was an undergraduate, experienced terrible anxiety whenever he had to write a paper for a specific course; it turned out that he thought the course ridiculous and the professor a fool, and was tempted to say so whenever he began writing. The paper required so much concentration and effort on his part precisely because he was working so hard *not* to say what he wanted to say in it, and was constantly apprehensive that he had in fact let some of his true feelings about the course and the professor leak out. The more he wanted to criticize this professor and his course, the more uneasy he grew. He wanted to do something—write a paper that would get him a good grade—and also wanted to insult his professor, and it was the latter that he put out of mind. Freud teaches us that what we put out of mind in this way comes back and bites us in the *derrière*, and the harder we try to keep it out of mind, the more insistently it returns and in the most surprising of ways. The harder my patient tried to write a paper that would convince his professor that he liked the class, took it seriously, and deserved a good grade, the more he felt blocked, couldn't write anything, or kept having to delete text that his fingers would end up typing, as if they had a mind of their own.

We can't say that he was unaware of his feelings about the professor or the course—he thought the professor a fool and the course ridiculous—but he was unaware of how those feelings were affecting his ability to write a paper for that professor. He was not conscious of those feelings while he was writing or even while he was complaining to me about his difficulty doing the assignment. And it didn't take much work on my part to elicit from him a pretty full description of his feelings. But at least while writing he was obviously attempting to push those feelings out of mind, and this led to a temporary form of writer's block.

Here is a somewhat more complicated example that Freud presents in his *Studies on Hysteria*. For many years, a woman whom Freud refers to as Emmy von N. (we'll just call her Emmy) involuntarily made a kind of clicking or clacking sound with her tongue whenever she was "excited." At the time, Freud was still practicing hypnosis, not having yet invented the technique that was to become known as psychoanalysis, and when he hypnotized Emmy this clicking was traced back to a moment at which she had been caring for her daughter, who had long been unable to fall asleep owing to a serious illness. When her daughter finally would fall asleep, Emmy "concentrated her whole willpower on keeping still so as not to awaken her." Freud then adds that, "Precisely on account of her intention [not to awaken her daughter] she made a 'clacking' noise with her tongue" (SE II, p. 5). When she recounted all the particulars of this first instance of clacking to Freud while hypnotized (along with a later instance), her somewhat minor symptom, which we might refer to today as a "nervous tic," disappeared for quite some time.

Today we would be inclined to hypothesize that the mother was aggravated and exasperated with this daughter whom she felt to be uncooperative, and that at least some part of her wished to punish the girl by waking her up again by making noise. Emmy knew full well that to do so would be *self-defeating*, as it would lead Emmy herself to further prolong her exhausting vigil by her daughter's bedside, yet something in her wanted to do it anyway (not being able to help but do things we know full well to be self-defeating is an important characteristic of neurosis). That is, we would hypothesize that Emmy was conflicted or of two minds: relieved her daughter had finally settled down and yet angry and/or frustrated at having been made to wear herself out at her bedside and wishing to lash out at her.

Why else would someone have to concentrate her willpower so diligently on not making any noise unless she was somehow tempted to make noise? Had no such punishing intention inhabited Emmy, there would have been no need for her to monitor herself or concentrate so hard on *not* making noise. This is a crucial, yet all-too-often overlooked facet of every instance of intense intentionality (or "trying so hard"): one has to focus one's attention so acutely precisely because something in one wants to do the opposite! If I have to be extra, extra careful not to miss an appointment, it is obviously because something in me does not want to go to it. If I have to be super careful not to put disparaging remarks about the professor in a paper I am writing for his course, it is because something in me wants to put the professor down. Trying too hard is symptomatic of a mind divided.

Later in his case study, Freud confirms our hypothesis about Emmy, for he tells us that "she had hated her child for three years" (SE II, p. 63), having had a whole series of "grievances against this child [who] had been very odd for a long time; she had screamed all the time and did not sleep, and she had developed a paralysis of the left leg which there had seemed very little hope of curing" (p. 60). At least one of the reasons why Emmy had hated this daughter for so long was that her beloved husband died suddenly right before her eyes while she was in bed, still weak from having given birth to this daughter. Although even the doctors were unable to revive her husband, Emmy somehow believed that "she might have been able to nurse her husband back to health if she had not been in bed on account of the child" (p. 63). Thus her fury at her daughter dated back almost to the very day of her birth.

She later told Freud that, although she had never been fond of the child, "no one could have guessed it from my behavior, for I did everything that was necessary" (p. 64); this suggests that she obliged herself to act a part that she did not feel, and no doubt resented the child still more because she forced herself to appear to be a good mother in the eyes of the world. This led her to doubly hate her daughter. (And the daughter undoubtedly picked up on this and perhaps even screamed and refused to sleep at least in part as a protest against what she considered to be her mother's unjust hatred of her.)

Thanks to Freud, it is elementary psychoanalytic thinking in our times to realize that people overemphasize or over-accentuate one thing because they mean the contrary. They say, "Oh, your outfit is *so* fab" when they find it atrocious. Or they say, "We would never even dream of hurting you" when that is *exactly* what they have in mind.

People are often led to work really hard to act one way precisely because they would like to act in the opposite way: they would like to insult their professor or annoy their child, but they strive as hard as possible not to. This usually leads to trouble, whether in the form of short-term writer's block or a tic (like making a clacking sound with one's tongue) that lasts for decades.

There are a number of different possible ways of describing what happens here: certain thoughts and feelings are shoved aside, put out of mind, or suppressed. Are they therefore "forgotten"? The student who wanted to insult his professor obviously had not forgotten them, but we might say he had overlooked or failed to realize the *link* between his thoughts about the course and his difficulty writing a paper for it. This is one way of talking about repression: *a fairly obvious link between two things is somehow broken or made to disappear.*

People often speak as though it is the feelings themselves that are repressed, but as we see here, my patient was quite aware of his feelings about the professor and the course. He just couldn't see any connection between those feelings and his writer's block. It was as if the obvious connection between the two was invisible to him or, assuming he had been aware of it at one point or another, as if the obvious connection had simply disappeared. The feelings continued to operate in his daily life, but he was unaware of the effect they were having.

Freud hypothesizes the following: our thoughts and feelings are usually connected to each other, but when repression occurs, what is repressed are, in one case, the thoughts (I forget, for example, my wishful thought about striking back at a parent who hits me), or, in the other case, the *link* between the thoughts and the feelings (not the feelings themselves).

Now different things may happen to feelings when repression of the thought related to them occurs (we will turn to what happens when the link is repressed in the next section):

1. They may be "suppressed" or pushed down, so to speak, and may find expression in occasional outbursts, when one is slightly or even considerably inebriated—in other words, when one lets one's guard down because one is exceptionally tired or one's inhibitions are muted owing to the effects of alcohol and/or drugs.

2. Feelings may be displaced. For example, instead of directly telling my professor I think he is a fool and his course is stupid, I call someone else a fool: maybe a fellow student in the class, the graduate assistant, or somebody else who reminds me in any way of the professor. To take a different example, let's say I have a girlfriend and I love her but sometimes she gets on my nerves, and she has in fact been getting on my nerves more and more as time goes by. We go to a bar together and some guy looks at her or looks at me in what I consider to be "the wrong way," and I get belligerent with him. My girlfriend is the one who is getting on my nerves, but I take it out on someone I don't even know rather than take it out on her. If you ask me afterward why I picked a fight with him, I'll give you all sorts

of reasons—I didn't like the way he was leering at my girlfriend, or I wasn't going to stand for the dirty looks he was giving me—but the fact remains that I probably would never have even noticed him if my girlfriend wasn't getting on my nerves. The anger I felt toward her but wouldn't allow myself to express to her was floating around in me, just looking for something to latch onto.

I might instead have gotten especially aggressive with my roommates, opponents on the tennis court, football players on a rival team, cashiers who charge me the wrong amount, or people who cut me off on the highway. But in all of these cases, the anger derives primarily from my relationship with my girlfriend, and not from the people I take it out on. Virtually everyone is familiar with the notion that when people are upset with someone in their family, they are sometimes led to "kick the dog." Why? Because the dog is less likely to hold it against you and make you pay for doing so than your family members are. Other people punch the wall, usually hurting themselves considerably in the process, and that's another example of what is known as the "displacement of affect." You want to punch someone, but instead of punching that person you punch the wall, or you want to hurt someone but instead of hurting that person you hurt yourself.

Being of two minds about something is, we have to assume, hard for most people. Love and hate are feelings that are hard to reconcile or live with simultaneously. So we tend to act as though only one of them exists at a time. If I am a ten or twelve year old, I may put the love I feel for a girl out of mind and tease her, make fun of her, pull her hair, and just generally act mean toward her. If I am older, I may put the hatred I feel toward her out of mind and bend over backwards to do everything I can think of for her, all the while harboring resentments that may one day show their face in a sudden outburst, betrayal, or breakup.

In many such cases, we find that a thought like "I hate so and so" is put out of mind, but the feeling persists and drifts until it finds a convenient outlet.

General schemas of repression

I mentioned earlier that, in the course of ordinary life experience, thought and affect usually go hand-in-hand. Let's say that I have uncharitable or even downright negative thoughts about my Uncle Bob because when

I was very young he once punished me harshly for doing something I didn't do. In most cases, those thoughts will be accompanied by feelings of revulsion toward him. Let us represent the initial situation in which thought and affect are connected as follows (with <—> signifying "link"):

$$\text{Thought} \longleftrightarrow \text{Affect}$$

Freud hypothesized that repression often acts by breaking the link between thought and affect; let us represent the subsequent situation in which thought and affect are disconnected owing to repression as follows:

$$\text{Thought} \parallel \text{Affect}$$

Repression, understood in this way, may lead to a wide variety of consequences:

1. The incident in which my uncle unjustly punished me may be forgotten, but my aversion to him remains; I loathe him, but I don't really know why, having forgotten what led me to despise him.

In this first instance, the memory of the incident or thoughts about his injustice have undergone repression, while their corresponding affect persists in consciousness. We may represent this as follows, where, once again, what is under the bar (or fraction-like line) is unconscious and what is above it is conscious:

$$\frac{\text{Affect}}{\text{Thought}}$$

In this instance, my affect strikes me as incomprehensible, and I may well latch onto some minor or unrelated incident to explain it to myself and others. Indeed, I may begin to find odious his religious beliefs, political convictions, profession, or lifestyle, and vehemently criticize all and sundry that espouse or practice them. I alight upon all kinds of reasons to criticize such beliefs and practices, and perhaps even formulate an entire counter-ideology to my uncle's, but my original impetus for doing so remains opaque to me (i.e., my feelings about the early events that involved my uncle have shifted to or become displaced onto his belief system or lifestyle). We might depict the situation here as follows, with Thought_1 representing my negative thoughts about my uncle owing to one or more events in my past, and Thought$_2$ representing my negative thoughts about certain religious beliefs, political convictions, professions, or lifestyles that I initially heard him express but that I may no longer even consciously associate with him:

$$\frac{\text{Thought}_2}{\text{Thought}_1} <\text{—}> \text{Affect}$$

We often see this sort of thing in young adults who become anarchists or Marxists and develop an elaborate critique of their parents' bourgeois lifestyles and of the society as a whole that they associate with their parents, whereas their beef at the outset was with their parents' failure to recognize them, give them credit and support for things they did, or love them enough. This is not to say that anarchism and Marxism don't have a lot to contribute, but that when certain people go into analysis, they become different sorts of leftists than they came in as, part of their motivation for critiquing bourgeois society having changed.

Another possible scenario that follows the same logic is one in which, rather than despising my uncle Bob, I begin to despise my brother Bob (who, let us suppose, was named after uncle Bob). The conflict in my mind that led me to forget what happened with my uncle does not exist in relation to my brother, and the affect that I formerly felt toward one Bob becomes attached to another Bob. We might refer to this, with Freud, as a "verbal bridge" or "switch word" (SE V, p. 341 n. 1), or simply as a "false connection"; or we might refer to it as a substitution of one Bob for another (or one signifier, S_2, for another signifier, S_1):

$$\frac{\text{Bob}_2}{\text{Bob}_1} <\text{—}> \text{Affect}$$

Note that both the quality and quantity of affect (in this case, extreme loathing) remain the same; it is merely the object of my loathing that has changed.

Yet another way in which repression may occur is as follows:

2. I do not remember the events that occurred that led me to loathe my uncle Bob, but I am always anxious around him, or develop a fear of being alone in a room with any man around his age.

In this instance, thoughts have been forgotten, and so as to ensure that they will not be remembered, the affect that had originally been associated with them (loathing) transmogrifies into something less tangible or legible: anxiety.

$$\frac{\text{Affect}_1}{\text{Thought}} \longrightarrow \text{Affect}_2$$

We might hypothesize that this kind of transformation of one affect into another occurs precisely when the thought is not entirely or thoroughly repressed and there seems to be a danger of my recalling what happened that initially made me loathe my uncle. On rare occasions, the transformation of affect goes so far that instead of abhorring him, I begin—strangely enough—to adore him; this is obviously the most perfect of disguises, which neither he nor I (nor virtually anyone else) can see through.

Repression may lead to yet another result:

3. I remember the event perfectly, but can't for the life of me recall how I felt about it at the time. Today I say, "So, it happened, no big deal: I never think about it." Where has the affect gone? Hard to say. Sometimes we see it in self-destructive behaviors, but it is not always easy to detect.

Yet another possible result is:

4. I remember nothing, nor do I feel angry in general or hate anyone, but I develop a facial tic, or move my head or arm in a curious way, whenever I am around a man who reminds me of uncle Bob; or I feel sick to my stomach and vomit whenever I am around any man who reminds me of him.

Here two different affects seem to be struggling for supremacy: a wish to attack uncle Bob and a will not to do so. The latter may be motivated in many different possible ways: I may wish to protect him from my own fury, perhaps at least in part because I also like him in some respects; I may wish not to show that I grant him any importance in my life; I may worry I will lose my parents' love if they catch me attacking my uncle or hear about it; I may believe that it is immoral to hit anyone and that I should be above all fits and displays of anger; and so on. Neither of my opposing affects seems to ever get the upper hand here, unlike the case of those people who seem to easily blow up at others, only to exhaust their anger fairly quickly and become more comfortable around them shortly after the explosion; we think of the latter as volatile and perhaps unpredictable, but they are rarely subject to symptom formation of the kind we see in those who never allow themselves to blow up in the first place.

Those who are forever at war with themselves end up expending huge quantities of their energy fighting their own tendencies, and to outside observers often seem quite dead, as if devoid of emotion (contemporary clinicians often characterize them as having "flat affect," overlooking the considerable affective forces that are warring within them). The tension they build up within themselves can, however, be quite self-destructive, leading to high blood pressure, muscular and skeletal problems, and—what is perhaps most common—the grinding of teeth. (Indeed, dentists are often the first professionals contacted by those who are fighting themselves in this way.) Self-destruction is tantamount, after all, to a kind of compromise, a compromise between the opposing forces that (1) wish to destroy another and that (2) seek to thwart any such violent activity. Instead of destroying others, I destroy myself.

By Way of Conclusion

It has often been noted regarding obsessives that they *recall* many important memories from their past, and can tell you about them in great detail, but without the slightest bit of emotion being attached to them; and regarding hysterics that they, on the contrary, *have forgotten* many important memories from their past but the feelings that were undoubtedly attached to them initially are still present in their lives or bodies, appearing in "crazy," incomprehensible ways insofar as they are detached from the thoughts and memories that gave rise to them.

In obsession we wonder where the emotion has gone—presumably into displaced objects of love or hatred, or into symptoms. In hysteria we know that the memories have been repressed, and that the affects have been set free to drift, alighting on this or that.

These are just a few of the many reasons Freud uncovered why people are not what they seem.

CASE DIS-MISS(ED)

CHAPTER 7

The slings and arrows of outrageous fortune

(A shorter version of this paper was presented in Zürich, Switzerland, at the invitation of Robert Langnickel, at the Lacan Seminar Zurich, on May 17, 2014.)

> *Between the imaginary relation and the symbolic relation lies the entire distance attributable to guilt. This is why, as psychoanalytic practice shows us, people always prefer guilt to anxiety.*
> —Lacan, 2013, p. 28

Today I will discuss the case of a middle-aged man who had been given a diagnosis of "major depressive disorder" by his two former therapists. It will, I think, be far more helpful to think of him in other diagnostic terms, but it was sadness and depression that were foremost in the patient's mind when he first came to see me.

I shall refer to this man, who grew up hearing and speaking both English and another language in his household, as J. He told me that he had been on antidepressant medications almost uninterruptedly since the age of twenty. He was, he reported, currently taking two antidepressants, an antianxiety medication, and sleeping pills. He had tried a dozen different antidepressants over the course of a decade and a half to no avail, since *he had never felt better on any of them*. But this did not dissuade him from taking them religiously.

Two years after beginning to work with me, he admitted that he had also been taking ibuprofen three times a day for twelve years (that is, since his mid-twenties) for aches and pains from weight training and aerobic exercise, in addition to a giant concoction of turmeric, magnesium, omega 3, and multivitamins—in all eleven vitamin supplements per day—to stave off aging, with which he was obsessed.

In addition to this rather potent chemical cocktail, he took tetracycline and used a variety of creams for dermatological problems (psoriasis, cystic acne, seborrhoeic dermatitis, and rosacea) and smoked marijuana regularly.

His first contact with me by email set the tone for what was to come, although I could not know it at the time. He wrote that he had been in therapy with two different therapists—one CBT and the other psychodynamic—over the past dozen years and would like to try a Lacanian approach, but could only afford 100 dollars per week. In the end, neither of his therapists was either CBT or psychodynamic in orientation, and he turned out to be among the wealthiest patients I have ever had, having inherited a considerable sum upon his father's death a few years prior to contacting me.[1] He did not, however, reveal this to me until seven months later when we went from three to four sessions a week.

Being what I generally refer to as a "therapy veteran"—that is, someone who had been in the psychiatric and psychotherapeutic system for a very long time—he had the story of his life down pat. At least it was the story as he liked to tell it to therapists and friends: his parents had been absolutely horrible to him, his mother having abandoned him to the evil clutches of his abusive, alcoholic father at around age six. He had been unloved by his mother and brutalized by his father—maybe even sexually abused by the latter (he initially professed to not be able to remember). And, the way he portrayed his childhood, it was a miracle that he was as "normal" as he appeared to be to most everyone today, he having heroically overcome his horrendous past. Although he once told me, "There's something fishy about that story," he liked to imagine he was a Jesus-like figure: as he put it, his mother had been victimized by his father, and she had offered up "her only son" in her stead (J is an only child). This made him into a true martyr, like St. Damien of Molokai, a saint who was revered by J's paternal grandmother.[2]

J claimed to feel terribly guilty—not for having in any way participated in or contributed to the mess of his childhood, adolescence, or adult life—but rather for not having *forgiven* his parents for what *they* did to him. He is from a Catholic background, had a sort of "religious conversion" to Catholicism in his mid twenties which led him to study theology for a while, and left his first therapist for a Jesuit counselor who echoed and encouraged the discourse of forgiveness. Thanks to that discourse, he was able to continue to completely misrecognize the reasons for his overwhelming feelings of guilt for many a year.

The misrecognition went so far that J even managed to interpret a somewhat vague comment made to him around age twenty by an aunt—to the effect that he should try to forgive himself—to mean that he should try to forgive himself, *not* for all the bad things he had done, but *for beating himself up* about not having pardoned his parents. He took it to mean that he should forgive himself for continuing to criticize himself for not having forgiven them. He concluded that his aunt's comment implied that he was not such a bad person after all, and did not deserve the punishment he had convinced her he had been inflicting upon himself.

When J revealed to his father in his early twenties that he felt guilty for how badly he had treated his college girlfriend, his father commented that one must not let oneself be brought down by guilt. This was construed by J as meaning that he had probably not done anything *that* awful, certainly nothing for which he could not be absolved. This allowed J to imagine that he was primarily guilty of stubbornly refusing to forgive himself.[3]

The religious discourse J adopted after his "conversion experience" to Catholicism fell on the unsympathetic ears of his first therapist, a psychiatrist who, like so many American therapists, was self-disclosive, telling J that he was an atheist. This led J to two-time the psychiatrist with another therapist, a Jesuit clinical social worker, who for six years indulged J's self-flattering discourse which allowed him to continue to see himself as something of a martyr: someone who was being tortured—albeit by himself—for crimes others had committed.

No punishment without a crime

Like most contemporary clinicians, J's therapists failed to heed Freud's warning in the case of the Rat Man about guilt, and about what is all too often characterized in our times as "inappropriate affect":

> When there is a *mésalliance* (misalliance) [...] between an affect and its ideational content (in this instance, between the intensity of the self-reproach and the occasion for it), a layman will say that the affect is too great for the occasion—that it is exaggerated— and that consequently the inference following from the self-reproach (the inference that the patient is a criminal) is false. On the contrary, the [analyst] says: "No. The affect is justified. The sense of guilt is not in itself open to further criticism. But it belongs to some other content, which is unknown (*unconscious*) and [must] be looked for. The known ideational content has only got into its current position owing to a false connection. We are not used to feeling strong affects without their having any ideational content, and therefore, if the content is missing, we seize as a substitute upon some other content which is in some way or other suitable, much as our police, when they cannot catch the [true] murderer, arrest [someone else] instead." (SE X, pp. 175–176)

In Freud's view, the Rat Man's guilty affect was not "inappropriate" but rather *displaced*. His self-recriminations and sense of being a criminal were connected to his long-standing wish that his father would die (his affect could thus be characterized as consonant with or "appropriate to" that wish), not to the fact that he was not present at the precise moment at which his father passed away.

A very similar misalliance was operative in the case of J. J's father had been hospitalized several times and J had taken a plane to go see him on each occasion. But the nth time his father sounded rather different on the phone, resigned and no longer fighting to stay alive. J asked his father if he should come see him and his father said "no," but he did not say so very emphatically. J indeed felt that this particular "no" meant "yes," but he nevertheless failed to go see his father in the hospital on this occasion.

The idea that the tremendous guilt he felt toward his father stemmed from the fact that he failed to go see him the time that it was not a false alarm but rather the real thing, was a "false [or spurious] connection." When J's therapists were tempted to downplay his guilt for having failed to do this as exaggerated or incommensurate, they should instead have been thinking *displacement*.[4]

My working assumption was that if J felt guilty, there must be some crime or crimes he felt he *had* committed, just not the one he was willing to admit to, which was the failure to forgive himself—something that I had never even heard referred to as a crime before. Although he sometimes mentioned that he felt good after abrupt scansions of sessions, he complained that it depressed him to sense that I was not on his side, by which he seemed to mean that I did not appear to believe his version of things, since I was always asking him to go further as if there were more there than met the eye.

Liar, liar, pants on fire[5]

In effect, I did not believe his version of things. In common parlance, J would be called a "pathological liar." Among the lies he repeatedly told people about his past were claims to have tried to commit suicide twice (this story was, as it turned out, inspired by the fact that his mother had once overdosed on Valium); claims to have been beaten up regularly by his father, whereas he was only occasionally slapped (after a year of analysis he admitted he had only been slapped perhaps ten times in his whole life, and he later reduced that figure to four or five); claims that his father only finally stopped drinking when J was twelve, whereas he stopped when J was nine;[6] and claims to have taken physical abuse from his father up until around age fifteen, at which point he pushed his father into a wall, his father then falling on his ass and never having struck J again—this event never actually occurred (it was a friend of J's who did this to that friend's own father, and J admired him for having done so). He often even pretended to have been sexually molested by his father, even though he knew it was a total fabrication.

J lied about virtually everything to women he wanted to become involved with, claiming, for example, to have been tested for HIV when he had not. He intentionally neglected to tell me he was still seeing both former therapists simultaneously when he first began to work with me. And he finally admitted to me after about a year that he had deliberately avoided talking to me about anything he considered to be too aggressive or perverse, even when it crossed his mind in session, because he had been entertaining the idea of coming to the university where I was teaching at the time to do a Ph.D. with me and wanted me to help him gain admission by writing him a strong letter of recommendation! (He obviously didn't realize that would have been impossible.)

J often lied to people he met, telling them that he was doing freelance translation work out of his home and teaching language classes at a local institute. And he would show up at a restaurant where he knew a lot of people with a good-looking woman whom he was not dating—she was just a friend—with the express intention of convincing the people there that he *was* dating her and was getting, as he put it, "plenty of sex."

On a couple of occasions, he even told me he had been thinking about committing suicide even though he had not, because he felt he did not have the "strength" to do psychoanalysis and wanted me to either tell him he was doing a great job or let him off the hook by allowing him to quit.

Most importantly, however, J told all of his therapists and anyone else who would listen that, after his mother kicked her husband out of the house because of his drinking when J was about three and a half, his mother didn't fight to retain custody of her son. He claimed that his father sued for custody just to piss his mother off (he was furious at her for having divorced him), not because he loved his son, and that his mother did not fight hard to keep him with her.

The story J told me for a long time was that his mother felt that she could not provide adequately for him, whereas his father and his father's family could give him a real home. There was only one bed in his mother's apartment (they were in a one-bedroom apartment at first and then in a studio apartment), and he and his mother were thus forced to share the same bed from around age three and a half, when his parents separated, until around age six when he went to live with his father. One of the clearest reasons his mother purportedly gave for "letting" J go live with his father was that in his father's apartment he would be able to have a room and thus a bed of his own.

In J's rendition of the story to me and everyone else, however, there was no room he could call his own at his father's place, because his father was temporarily living with his own parents, the father's business having gone bankrupt. Later it came out that there *was* indeed an extra room in the paternal grandparents' apartment for him, but that J *preferred* to sleep in his father's bedroom with his father. They slept in his mother and father's former conjugal bed, J sleeping on what used to be his mother's side of that bed. Being in that spot made him feel like a *whore* in relation to his father, as did his willingness (and indeed eagerness) to take his father's money, which J perceived his mother to do as well, both before and after the divorce. This lends special salience to J's favorite way of complaining about how badly he is feeling: "I've been feeling *hor*rible," he regularly whines, placing special emphasis on the *whore* in *horrible*. (He doesn't pronounce it "har-rible," as many Americans do, but "whore-able.") One of his extreme ways of formulating his mother's behavior was to say that his mother had long been a victim of the father's angry drunken treatment and that she had offered her son up to be a kind of sacrificial lamb. The idea seemed to be that the father would now satisfy his aggressive impulses with J and stop harassing J's mother, who couldn't take any more of the father's anger.

The reasons for the change in custody seemed for a long time to be the biggest lie J had ever told the whole world and himself as well.

"Abandonment"

The time J spent alone with his mother between three and a half and six was initially presented to me as "heaven on earth," he and his mother rivaling in their pillow talk to say which of them loved the other one more. ("I love you." "No I love you." "Well, I love you more.") Later it became clear that, even at that tender age, J already felt things were a little too intense between himself and his mother. One day, his mother teased him about a girl he had a crush on in kindergarten, and he immediately felt obliged to call the girl a whore, as if he felt he had to prove to his mother that he was exclusively devoted to her, not to the girl at school. (He did, however, see his father on weekends between three and a half and six.)

At age six or seven, he attended a wedding and realized that if he ever got married he would have to kiss his bride in front of his mother (and father), which struck him as impossibly embarrassing. This would be to admit that he loved a woman other than mom, whereas up until that point he had been cheating, as it were, on his mother with his father and vice versa.

J's account of the change in custody that occurred when he was around six years of age was extremely vague at first. Although his mother had purportedly kicked his father out due to alcoholism, feeling him to be unfit as a husband, and the father had not yet stopped drinking, she apparently immediately gave in to her ex-husband's request for full custody of J.

In the tiniest of dribs and drabs, a fuller picture of the situation came into focus. It turned out that the mother had given the father six months to stop drinking, but he had not stopped and so she asked him to leave. After they separated, the father, who was still as in love as ever with J's mother, bullied her by always sending his child support checks late, knowing full well that she had virtually no other means of support. She apparently did fight to retain custody of J for quite some time, but was eventually worn down by the father's repeated withholding of money.

A time even came before the change in custody when she asked J himself, at around the age of six, who he would prefer to live with, his mother or his father. J had been seeing his father on weekends and seemed to be very much enjoying his stays with his father and the father's family, a fact he made plain to his mother. To this day, J claims that he cannot recall what he said in reply to his mother's question, only that he felt torn.

In retrospect, he came to feel it was totally unfair of her to have asked the question and to have placed such a choice in the hands of a six year old who couldn't possibly have known what was good for him. When these details finally came out, he admitted he had *knowingly* lied to me about all of this for four years!

After yet another year of analysis, he recalled an incident that occurred when he was around five years old: he was supposed to spend the night at a friend's house while his mother had a man she was interested in over for dinner—it was to be her first date in ages. Feigning illness (or anxiety?), he called her shortly after the man was to arrive and begged her to come pick him up and bring him home. "You ruined my night," she told him angrily as she did so. In the analysis, he told me that her reaction made him feel unloved or at least less loved than the man with whom she had the date, and that he decided at that point to make her feel the same thing—unloved. Soon afterward, he began telling her how much fun he had with his father on the weekends, that it was more fun to be at his house than at hers, and eventually that he wanted to go live with his father.

Still later, J came to realize that his sense of feeling rejected and abandoned by his mother probably stemmed from identification with his father, for his father felt rejected and abandoned by the mother who had long threatened to kick him out of the house owing to his alcoholism and had finally done so. In a sense, for J to feel abandoned by his mother was a form of solidarity with or identification with his father.

Even later it came out that the feeling of having been abandoned by his mother may actually have first come from having been left by a nanny who took care of him as a toddler while his mother was indisposed for five months. It seemed that his mother had perhaps taken the blame, in his mind, for the nanny's departure.

Amid the constant stream of reproaches he leveled at his mother in his own head over the better part of two decades, an involuntary thought came to him one day after about fifteen months of analysis: "I've been blessed with a really great mother." After telling me about that thought in a session, he noticed that his face had turned bright red and he wet his bed that night.

J's face is often very red—a condition for which he has received several different diagnoses and treatments—and he associates this with shame (being red-faced) and anger, feeling that others can see anger written all over his face, which he feels must scare them away. Red, irritated skin has been one of his major complaints since the beginning of our work together.

On another occasion, after purportedly being angry at himself for twenty-four hours because he had not told his mother he hated her when he had spoken with her at length on the phone, he admitted to loving her intensely and hating feeling that he wasn't loved in return by her with the same intensity, even though at the same time he knew that he was. He described his anger at his mother as "the most intense feeling" he'd ever had—but clearly the same could be said of his love for his mother.

Returning to the more usual blame game, J told me that if his mother had really and truly loved him, *she should have paid no attention to what he said at six years of age*—implicitly admitting thereby that he had told her he wanted to live with his father. She should have fought to keep him at any cost. If she had kicked his father out for being an alcoholic, how could she have possibly delivered her son into the hands of such a sick man? (She apparently believed alcoholism to be a sickness.) Either she had proven herself to be a *hor*rible mother by doing so (being willing to sacrifice him in her own stead) or she had proven that J himself was insufficiently lovable.

He decidedly favored the first option in this alternative. Indeed, he acted as though he were God's gift to the world, better than everyone else, and entitled to special treatment from one and all. Nevertheless, in many of his long-term relationships with women, he had done everything possible to test the woman's love for him by treating her abominably, using her sexually in ways he considered to be thoroughly degrading, accusing her of not loving him, and—if that wasn't enough to chase her away—pretending to have cheated on her.

Putting love to the test

J seemed to be dead set on forcing a woman to multiply proofs of her love for him, and the most enduring of the trials he would put a woman through was his so-called erectile dysfunction ("ED"). Once he began antidepressant medication, he had a ready excuse for his erectile problems, it being well known that antidepressant medications depress libido, but his impotence began well before he started taking such drugs.

Since Lacan tells us in Seminar VIII that the phallus is essential to comedy,[7] I will not resist the temptation to repeat one of the funniest stories J recounted related to his erectile difficulties. After telling me a long, elaborate story about what he believed to be the first occasion upon which he had had problems getting and maintaining an erection, he made an *incidental remark*, as if changing the subject, that he had never mentioned before about something he saw in a girls' dormitory during his freshman year at college. Several girls he knew shared an apartment in the dorm and on their living room wall he saw a poster which was a chiastic takeoff on a well-known expression: "A good man is hard to find." The poster in the girl's apartment showed a handsome man with big muscles, and the caption, borrowed from Mae West, was: "A hard man is good to find." The analysand commented that he concluded upon seeing the poster that *"that was what women really wanted."*

Several years prior to his freshman year he had been lifting weights in order to have a "hard body." Since seeing the poster, however, he had stopped lifting weights and stopped getting hard with women. In prior sessions we had discussed the possibility that he was in some way determined *not* to give women what they wanted, just as he was determined to frustrate his mother's requests and wishes. He agreed that something of that kind seemed to be going on, but he could not understand how or why, so it remained somewhat abstract to him. In this session we were able to establish with pretty good confidence that he saw this poster shortly before his first problem getting and maintaining an erection that was not alcohol-related. Believing he now knew exactly what women wanted, he knew exactly how *not* to give it to them!

The proximate cause of his erectile problems was thus established to be his wish to deprive women of something, to disappoint them, to *not* be what he thought they wanted him to be. Why he wished that was a far more encompassing question, but the *incidental* remark about the poster at least allowed a connection to be made between his so-called erectile dysfunction and the kick he got out of frustrating and disappointing women, both of which seemed to go to the core of his way of relating to them. He would rather forgo sexual jouissance with the women he dated—reserving that for masturbation to Internet porn—to obtain another kind of jouissance, an unavowable satisfaction in making women unhappy (he even admitted that he enjoyed seeing signs of suffering in their faces). He mentioned that he obstinately refused to take Viagra in order to be able to have an erection with a woman (even though he took all kinds of other pills). Indeed, he hoped that a woman would be hurt and insulted when he couldn't get it up with her, for she would think that there must be something wrong with her or that she was not good-looking enough to excite him. In this sense, to him failure was success: to fail to get an erection was to succeed in hurting a woman.[8]

Work is a four-letter word

This was not the only sense in which failure amounted to success in his view.

J has rarely worked at anything, other than thwarting his father's wishes and his therapies, and went so far on one occasion as to actually say, regarding his studies, that "failure is success"[9]—for his poor academic performance annoyed his father greatly—and on another occasion as to say that being depressed "is a [fulltime] job"! (One might well wonder who he was doing that job for.) He was most depressed during the work day, not at night. During the daylight hours, he felt he should be working, that his father would want him to be working. He admitted that he wasn't actually depressed for the six years he did hold down a job, but that didn't stop him from taking antidepressant medications during that time.

One girlfriend of his even complained that he made her do all the work during sex. His conviction is that women always dupe him with their attractiveness and then demand a million orgasms. His response is, "No, not a single one." Commenting one day that a woman must not ask him to make her climax with his penis, he added, "My penis has no work ethic" (a rather damning statement in a country like the United States!).

J hated it when a woman showed sexual desire, for if she was horny it was not really for him, it was just for a penis, which meant that it could be anyone's penis. He wanted to be wanted and loved for his subjective difference from everyone else, not for what he shared with all men. He detested all expressions of women's sexual desire and jouissance, and put women through a kind of test: if they really wanted him to perform, he couldn't. If, however, they just wanted to be with him and didn't care if they could have sex with him, then he could perform. If they didn't want it they could have it; if they did, they couldn't.

In his own mind, he was testing them to see if their love for him was unconditional; if they were willing to forego sex, then they loved him like a mother would love her child, and he could play the part of a baby with them.[10] He often seemed to believe that all women wanted from him was sex (and money), probably because at one level all he wanted from them was sex. This was because he believed that *real men* only want sex from women, not love (a real man's motto is "love 'em and leave 'em," he opined), and that he had to prove that he was a man by focusing so much, at least in his talk with other men, on sex. Men should be "heartbreakers," not momma's boys.

Above all, though, he craved to be loved, and came to think of a woman's willingness to have sex with him as a sign of love if and only if she didn't enjoy it very much. Her not enjoying it would serve as proof that she was doing it primarily for him, not for her own sexual satisfaction. Women's sexual satisfaction scared J—as it does many men—at least in part because he felt that it implied that women were primarily with him for their own enjoyment, not because they loved him. If he felt that with a specific woman, then it seemed to him that it was his erect penis she was after, and that was the very thing he would not provide.

Who's the boss?

With male peers his attitude always seemed to flip-flop between domination and submission. He would invent stories to make himself look good and pretend he had read all kinds of things he had never read to sound as though he were better than everyone else, all the while thinking himself far more inadequate than most of his friends.

He often would not even notice that a specific woman existed until he heard she was involved with a male friend of his; then he would anxiously pursue her until he seduced her. He would nervously think about the other man from whom he had stolen the woman or on whom he had gotten her to cheat, seeming to get a great deal more juice out of the rivalry with this other man than out of the relationship with the woman herself. As Freud indicates, many men need to feel jealous of and have "gratifying impulses of rivalry and hostility" toward the other man, the man who was already involved with the woman before he came on the scene.[11]

Some of the triangles J got himself into were quite complex, and in one case J was slapped around by an outraged boyfriend. This gave him pause for thought, although he believed he deserved it. But it did not put a crimp in his style, since he continued to repeat the same kind of behavior for many years. He was far more interested in angering other men than in a woman's desire for him or even in his desire for her. He would spend a great deal of time imagining that the men whose women he had seduced wanted to kill him, and he would get very worked up about it. Consciously he was incredibly "stressed out" by this, but clearly he derived a kind of rivalrous jouissance from it.

With men, this sort of imaginary, rivalrous jouissance predominated, and with women he sought out unconditional love for himself (while showing them no love and giving them no sexual enjoyment). When there was no other man present in a woman's life, he would feel jealous of her relationship with her father.

J's relationship to the medical establishment as Other with a capital O was revealed in the curious way he spoke about decreasing the dosage of psychiatric medications he took as he weaned himself from them; he repeatedly said that he was "going down on" the meds. "Going down on" is a well-known idiomatic expression for performing oral sex on someone, and he spoke as if he were giving oral sex to the medication or to the medical establishment itself every time he took a pill or shaved a milligram off a pill with a razor blade in an effort to reduce the dose.

He explicitly said he felt that the entire medical establishment was "fucking [him] up the ass" by feeding him pills, sticking them in his mouth—even though he was the one who requested them right from the outset and repeatedly for most of two decades. He requested his first anti-anxiety medication simply because a girlfriend of his was taking one and he couldn't stand the idea that she would be happier than he was; and he went on an antidepressant because he was eager to embrace the idea that depression was a disease, a disease he could blame on his father, imagining that he had inherited it from his father.

Nevertheless, he preferred to think the medications were forced or foisted upon him. He even had a kind of obsession with looking at his mouth, thinking that the area between his mouth and nose looked like part of a vulva. By feeding him pills, psychiatrists were screwing him as though he were a submissive woman.[12]

Desperately seeking punishment

Perhaps the clearest manifestation of his beef with the Other with a capital O was the fact that, although he had plenty of money, he never paid any of his bills on time, hoping that representatives of the telephone company, the electric company, and credit card companies would come after him and punish him (like the boyfriends of girls he seduced). He was constantly having his services disconnected and having to go to great lengths to get them reconnected. He surprised himself one day by saying, "If I don't pay, they'll cut off my …" Lapsing into silence for a moment as he realized what he had been about to say, he exclaimed, "Holy Jesus!"

Later on in the analysis, he proffered that he delayed paying his bills to awaken in the Other a will to dominate him, the Other taking the form of father substitutes here. "When I feel dominated," he said, "I feel I exist."

J would get several parking tickets a week and hoped to be pulled over and mightily fined for such infractions. On numerous occasions his car was booted, because he had hundreds of unpaid parking tickets, or towed because it was illegally parked. His finest moment, so to speak, was being forced to spend the night in jail for driving without insurance or registration.

His relationships with older men have always been incredibly fraught. He held a job for six years (prior to inheriting money from his father), and arrived at work late every day, feeling (or hoping that his boss would feel) that he was so wonderful they could not possibly fire him. He seemed, in a way, to be daring his boss to fire him.

He never paid his taxes and refused to show up for jury duty, which made him incredibly anxious as he anticipated being punished for these mostly minor crimes. He was lucid enough to have told me on one occasion that were he to pay his bills, taxes, parking tickets, and my fee too in a timely fashion, he would be no better off, for he would still feel anxious and guilty but have nothing *specific* to feel guilty for!

If he could feel guilty for these minor crimes, perhaps he could avoid reckoning with the far more major crimes he obviously believed he had committed: deliberately making life difficult for his father; doing everything possible to piss his father off and disappoint him, even when J was dimly aware that J was disappointed in or angry at himself (e.g., for performing poorly in a fencing tournament at age eleven); systematically disobeying his father's rules and lying to him; wishing both of his parents dead; and throwing his father's money out the window by flunking out of one college program after another, incurring huge fines for failure to pay bills and parking tickets, and even paying for services never rendered by missing sessions with me. After some six years of analysis, he indicated that he believed he himself had killed his father little by little by frustrating and angering him, "slowly eroding" his father's health.

The anxiety and tension he felt about the minor crimes struck him as just like the anxiety and tension he felt while growing up with his father. J had played guitar for a couple of years around puberty at the instigation of one of his father's girlfriends but had soon grown tired of it. When he realized that his father heartily disapproved of rock musicians and their music, he embraced the guitar and rock music wholeheartedly, saying that he thrived on the rift this created between himself and his father, adding that the tension he thrived on at that time later turned into depression.

One of his greatest pleasures in life was to annoy his father, and he had been missing that sorely since his father's death a few years prior to beginning analysis. He even reported that he felt that his life had somehow ended when his father died, and that he was living as though he were already dead and looking back on his life. His father seemed to him to be omnipresent and omniscient now that he was dead. Whenever J was masturbating, he—like the Rat Man—imagined his father watching him.[13]

J was quite cognizant at some level that his whole life project was to say "fuck you" to his father and to deliberately avoid accomplishing anything; his whole stance was negative, "telling the Other to fuck off," as he put it. What was most precious to him in life was to blame his mother and his father for being *hor*rible parents, and he felt that were he to be successful or happy in any way whatsoever, he would be letting both of them off the hook. This he absolutely refused to do, all the while feeling like a terrible criminal for not doing so, since he was simultaneously aware of his parents' good qualities and the many nice things they had done for him. He refused to allow them to feel good about themselves or to in any way enjoy his successes. In a word, his battle cry was, "The Other shall never get any satisfaction from me!"

He wanted to be completely consumed by anger at his father for taking him away from his mother: his father would have to pay forever. Being in a depressed mood was designed, J told me, to have an effect on his father—J would always blame his poor grades, which annoyed his father no end, on his depression. In the first years of his analysis, his sadness and depressed mood were designed, he said, to have an effect on me, to make me feel guilty and do something. As he put it, "My mood is my grossest symptom," felicitously including a double meaning in the formulation.

After about a year of analysis J revealed to me that the beginning of my *Clinical Introduction to Lacanian Psychoanalysis*, which he had read prior to contacting me, had baited him: it was as if I were saying he was enjoying his symptom and that infuriated him; he refused to believe it. He began analysis with me in order to challenge me: "Let's see what you can do—you're not going to be able to change me!" "You might even make me worse."[14]

Simultaneously, he imagined that I might make things so bad for him that he would reach a breaking point at which "something would be released." Then he might be able to "walk out the door and not feel the depression anymore," as if a stupid blunder on the Other's part could once and for all relieve him of guilt, sadness, and depression. But he slipped as he said this, and instead uttered, "walk out the door and not *feed* the depression anymore."

After making that slip, he wondered whether I would conclude he was a fraud and refuse to work with him anymore. If I did, he would have won, for I would have admitted that I couldn't change a fraud like him who knowingly "fed" his own depression.

His whole reason for starting psychoanalysis, he told me, was in order to be able to rival with me, compete in a kind of "chess match." "I'm in analysis because I don't know whether it works,"[15] making it clear that he wanted to prove that it doesn't.

Guilty pleasures

The degree to which guilt permeated J's existence was attested to by his attitude when awaiting the results of blood tests: "I feel like I'm waiting for a guilty/not guilty verdict." If the doctors told him he had a fatal illness, he would have to reckon with the notion that he was guilty for having wanted his parents dead, for example, indeed for wanting everyone dead.

He believed that he was "a moral monster." When he cowardly lied to someone, instead of saying what he thought and expressing what he wanted, he felt guilty and depressed. He hated people who blamed everything on others, because they took no responsibility for themselves. Yet he felt he was a "pussy," like his father who he felt had been "pussy-whipped" by his mother and by his second wife. (Nevertheless, his father seemed strong and phallic to J when he was angry.) He felt that both he and his father were deficient in courage. "I am exactly the type of person I don't like." "I think of myself as a lie."

He was convinced that if he was suffering, it was—as in the Old Testament—because he had done something wrong (when the people of Israel were suffering, it was because one or more of them had committed a crime against God). In a dream he reported, he had been "sentenced to death," his crime being clear. His depression was a message (from God about his guilt? Or to his father: "See how unhappy you've made me!"), not an illness. He had, he said, "tons of evil in [his] heart."

Nevertheless, his motto was "Never forgive!" The flip side of this was that he wanted to be forgiven by his father who did have a good side and who J devoted himself to angering; he admitted to taking his father's "less than ideal parenting as some sort of *hor*rific crime." J wanted to be forgiven "for all the trouble [he] caused and all the money [his father] spent on [him]" and "for wanting [his father] dead." The problem, as J saw it, was that it was too late now for him to be forgiven by his father.

A change in subjective position

When, after a year and a half of analysis, J began to experience what he called "random glimpses of joy," he found it hard to accept that he might not be depressed. After about four years of analysis, he stopped taking the very last medication he had been taking and commented, "To not take a pill is to say I don't have an illness." He indicated that he had a lot riding "on the idea of being sick" and that it was difficult to give it up.

He had created an impossible situation in which he couldn't win: to be happy was to make his parents happy, which he refused to do. If he was miserable, his parents would be miserable too. But he simultaneously felt his father preferred it when J was miserable, frowning at his smiles, laughter, and high spirits—so to be miserable was to give his father what he wanted (or so he wanted to believe), and he couldn't do that either! "I've created a circular, impossible situation," he admitted. "What would it be like to let all of this go?"

To let go of his father would be to stop blaming him and more generally to stop blaming the past and using it to make himself look like a hero. But that would imply, J said, that he would have to do something, achieve something in the present, in order to look good to other people. There lay the rub!

Achieving something in the present was much harder to do, and J's unwillingness to strive to succeed at something resonates with Lacan's comments in *Television*, which I will do my best to translate as follows:

> People qualify sadness as depression by basing it on the soul [...]. But it is not an emotion [*état d'âme*: literally, state of the soul], it is simply a moral failing [*faute*: crime, fault, misconduct, offense, wrongdoing], as Dante, and even Spinoza, put it: a sin, which implies moral cowardice, which in the final analysis can only be situated on the basis of thought—that is, on the basis of the duty to put it well [*bien dire*] or to find one's way around in the unconscious, in structure. (1974, p. 39)

With terms like moral failing, cowardice, and sin, Lacan seemingly brings us back to the religious language with which J so dearly wanted to understand his inaction in life. But Lacan manages to turn it on its head: instead of a failure to forgive, Lacan points to a lack of courage to live, a dearth of the guts to face the thoughts, desires, and drives by which one is inhabited.

How the analysand can be inspired to have the courage to live and face all of that is another story. Psychiatrists, who have mostly sold *their souls* to the pharmaceutical companies, are eager to convince people they are victims of their "chemical imbalances," their "damaged brains," and many patients are anxious to be so convinced, to be told their problems are not of their own making. Psychologists are often eager to convince people they are victims of their upbringing, and side with their patients against their patients' parents and relatives who are viewed as unadulteratedly evil.

Given the current view in the U.S. that we are all victims, it is no easy matter to interest people in talk therapy, and even once they are in it to guide them to a point—an unpredictable, unfathomable point—where they "decide" to do something for themselves (see Whitaker, 2010, p. 125), find the will to do something to get out of what they've spent decades getting into. As one patient put it, "depression is like a weed that I have been watering, and I want to pull up that weed" now by the roots (p. 150).[16]

One might think here of Lacan's "unsoundable [or unfathomable] decision of being" ("*insondable décision de l'être*"; *Écrits*, p. 145), even if it was formulated in the context of psychosis. And I would add that this decision to be something other than an object or victim is not made once and for all, but must be made again and again as each unpleasant memory is unearthed, as each unsavory wish and "filthy enjoyment" is faced.

Transference matters

Before turning to diagnosis, let me briefly comment on how J situated himself in relation to me in the transference over the course of the first seven years of the analysis.

As I mentioned earlier, he at one point said, "I'm in analysis because I don't know whether it works." He clearly wanted, at some level, to prove that psychoanalysis doesn't work. He admitted to having been attracted to psychoanalysis from the outset because he thought it meant people have no free will—indeed, no will whatsoever—and therefore he wouldn't have to try to do anything to change. He believed that, theoretically speaking, psychoanalysis freed him from all responsibility for his life. If he was going to change in the course of his analysis, it would be up to his analyst to make him do so. He himself wouldn't have to make any effort—I would somehow change him for him, as though I were performing some kind of medical operation on him.

Nevertheless, he clearly saw me as like his father at first, and thought of his entering into analysis as a big challenge to me and to psychoanalysis as a whole—you will not change me, just go ahead and try! No matter what his father did, he wasn't going to change J, and psychoanalysis wasn't going to either. He would prove them both impotent, which presumably would then make him feel more potent.

In the course of the first year of our work together, he expressed quite a bit of aggression toward me, and made it clear that he did not want to dream, associate, or work in any analytic way whatsoever. When he did occasionally recall a dream, he would often wait for a few days or even a week before recounting it to me. When I asked him why, he admitted that it was because he did not want me to be able to make much of his dreams and believed that if he waited long enough, he would forget most of the prior day's events, which would make free association less fruitful. He indicated that he felt that I did not sympathize with him and that I was not "on his side." He at times claimed to want me to empathize with his plight, but actually seemed to do just fine without me doing so; he nevertheless complained about my perceived lack of empathy. (He once commented that he and his father were alike in that they were both utterly devoid of empathy.)

He slept through many sessions, no matter how late in the morning or afternoon we scheduled them, and he often would not pick up the phone when I called him to find out whether he was coming or not.

He often referred to my "scanding him"—this was related to the ending of our variable-length sessions—as though he clearly experienced it as some kind of castration. He indicated that he often wanted to snap at me, yell at me. After seven months, he came to feel that he was not paying me enough money per session and, when we moved from three sessions per week to four, finally admitted that he had more money than he had initially said.

He clearly identified with me as someone he thought of as intelligent. After a year of analysis, he reported that he had had some sort of momentary "supernatural experience of total love" for me, feeling at one with me, saying that it was orgasmic and oceanic. Whatever it was (identification with some sort of authority figure?), it certainly was fleeting.

After about a year and a half of analysis, he began occasionally coming to sessions high on marijuana. This largely subsided at the point at which, one day when he revealed that he had smoked pot before coming to the prior session, I said something like, "As if you thought I couldn't tell?" This disturbed him, as he seemed to want to believe that I could not tell when he was high, and he grilled me for details as to how I could tell. I supplied a few, to the effect that he was often incoherent and seemed unable to remember what he had said from one moment to the next; he contested this, asserting that he remembered everything in sessions when he was high, but soon stopped getting stoned before sessions. The enjoyment in doing so very likely had something to do with thinking he was pulling the wool over my eyes, and taking a kind of secret enjoyment for himself without my knowing about it. The fact that I did know made such secret enjoyment impossible.

After about two years, J would occasionally pretend he was extremely depressed in order to get me to say something, to show him a sign of love and tell him he was doing a good job in psychoanalysis. I never told him any such thing, naturally, but I would sometimes offer extra sessions the same day when he seemed to be extremely depressed, which served in a sense to "call his bluff," extra sessions not being what he wanted from me. At that time he would sometimes admit that his mood was designed to affect me, to make me feel guilty so that I would make an exception for him, or do something special for him.

After over two years of analysis, he finally admitted exactly how much money he had inherited from his father. He said at that point that he felt he should be paying me more but refused to do so; this, too, made him feel like a criminal.

After almost three years of analysis, he would get angry at me when I would intervene or interpret something: "I'm paying you to sit there and listen to me whine endlessly," he exclaimed. At that point in time, the only thing he was willing to work hard at was thwarting the analysis.

After three and a half years, he told me that he had read in my *Clinical Introduction to Lacanian Psychoanalysis* that I call patients when they do not show up for sessions; he thought he could get me to chase him right from the get-go, just like the cable, phone, electric, and other companies.

At various points he averred that he sometimes hoped to anger me, for if I were to get really angry at him, he would take it as a sign of love. I could only be so angry at someone I really cared about.

For the past few years, he has never missed a session, and now rarely arrives late for sessions. He requests extra sessions himself when he is upset about something, recalls dreams with some regularity (even if he sometimes still waits for a few days before recounting them to me), and works quite hard at his analysis, the analysis clearly having become the most important undertaking in his life. Even though he still occasionally thinks he sees some resemblance to his father in my face, most of the aggressive and challenging transference related to his father has subsided. Curiously enough, he once recently called his mother "by accident" when he meant to call me—might that be a harbinger of things to come?

Diagnosis

In mentioning the case of the Rat Man a couple of times earlier on, I may have given the impression that I wish to argue that J is an obsessive neurotic. Although one can find many traits of obsession in his life story, I would argue that his positioning of himself as object *a* suggests instead a diagnosis of hysteria. He positions himself vis-à-vis his mother as an object that can be lost and that he imagines being lost in a number of different ways; and he positions himself vis-à-vis his father as his father's "bitch." As he once put it, he went from being his mother's "darling" to being his "father's prostitute."

Let us consider first his position with respect to his father. J was certainly struck by his own willingness (indeed, perhaps, by his eagerness) to take his mother's place in the conjugal bed—the bed his parents had slept in together as long as they lived together—when he moved in with his father at age six. Recall that another bedroom had been available in the grandparents' apartment, but that J had preferred to share his father's bed, rather than live and sleep in his own room. He referred to himself in this context as his father's "bitch," and used the same exact term when he talked about his willingness—and, indeed, eagerness—to take his father's money, just like J's mother did. J came to conclude, at least in part, that women slept with men in order to enjoy their money, and that they were willing to do almost anything and put up with almost anything in order to get that money.

In addition to thinking of himself as his father's bitch, he also devoted a great deal of energy to getting a rise out of his father, and to trying to elicit punishment from his father. He would deliberately do many things that he knew his father would disapprove of and/or be furious about, one of which was to masturbate in his father's bed as an adolescent, rather than going into the bathroom. He was, as he put it, always "anxious" that his father would walk in while he was doing so, obviously at some level wanting his father to walk in.

J did drugs that his father openly disapproved of; he studied as little as possible; he began playing electric guitar when he heard his father disapprove of it (his father only liked classical music and wanted him to play the violin); and J fervently wanted to pursue a career in music until his father acquiesced and said that he could try his hand at it, at which point J no longer seemed to have much enthusiasm for practicing. In short, the lion's share of J's activities in life were aimed at eliciting his father's disapproval and wrath. He often was excited at the possibility of being punished by his father and was disappointed if his father did not evince a will to punish him. On the one occasion when his father actually apologized to him for having yelled at him about something—accusing him for having moved something that he had not in fact moved—J felt that apology to be a sign of weakness and disliked it intensely. He seemed to need to see his father as a strong man, and J orchestrated things in such a way as to incite his father to dominate him. Indeed, J viewed virtually all relationships—whether amicable, sexual, or psychoanalytic—as essentially involving a dominator and a submissive party, he being the latter on most occasions.

He lived in a state of constant tension and anxiety, always looking to provoke an authority figure and only relieved of tension and anxiety when punished. When telephone companies, utilities, credit card companies, and the police would come after him and force him to pay his bills or get insurance for his car, he would feel that all was once again well with the world: everything was back in its proper place. The whole time he was delaying payments or not insuring his car, which would often last for months, he was in a state of heightened tension and constant anxiety, which only getting drunk or stoned could assuage.

We could formulate his relationship to the Other with a capital O, in particular to male authority figures, as one in which he wished to elicit a furious will to punish on their part, he being the object a that their fury revolved around. Such positioning allowed him to bring out the lack in the Other—that is, a desire in the Other for things to be different, a desire that J be a certain way and not another: $(a \lozenge \cancel{A})$. This is the formula for hysteria, as Lacan presents it in Seminar VIII (pp. 294 and 300), and the bringing out of a desire (which proves the existence of a lack) in the Other allows the subject to know who and what he is as a precious, albeit ofttimes hated object of the Other's desire.

Some of these details might incline us to think more of perversion—and of masochism, more specifically—than of hysteria, but my sense is that J's aim was not to bring out anxiety in the Other and be the one pulling the strings of their interactions (see Fink, 1997, chapter 9), but rather to prop up the Other by provoking evidence of the Other's will and power. A few biographical incidents (one involving an animal, one an infant, and another a toddler; J referred to these as his "darkest moments") were suggestive of sadism, as was his treatment of numerous women, but my general sense is that he primarily held tension and anxiety within himself, rather than casting it upon others. Rather than focusing the lion's share of his energy on bringing out the castration in others, he seemed to dwell and at times even wallow in his own. Even as he tried to convince others he was sexually potent and highly well-read, he was acutely aware of his deficiencies in those areas. On a couple of occasions, J tried to get me to admit I'd made a mistake by saying something to him that he believed I shouldn't have said, but he virtually never seemed to try to make me anxious or cast his own castration onto me, as we would expect to see were he perverse.

Let us turn now to J's positioning with respect to his mother. When, in talking in analysis about his mother's health and advanced age, he would mention "[his] mother's loss," he would often become quite confused about the meaning of these words: was it J himself who would lose his mother or was it his mother who would lose J? "The loss of [his] mother" was a frequent theme for many years, and he would always evince perplexity about what he himself meant by the expression. It seemed that no matter how clearly the context implied that he was talking about his mother's inevitable death at some point in the next ten or so years, something in him was always more concerned with what it would mean to her to lose him—whether figuratively or literally. Figuratively, he would often contemplate in his mind "breaking up with [his] mother," and at one point in the analysis told her over the phone that he didn't love her, speculating that it would kill her to hear such a thing—which it didn't, even if it hurt her and brought her to tears. Literally, he would imagine what would happen if he were to die in a plane crash, especially in a plane crash that occurred when he was on his way to visit her. Again his thoughts about dying in a plane crash did not focus on what he himself would miss out on in life, but on what the effect would be on his mother to have her only son suddenly taken away from her.

As amazingly attached as he was to her, which might allow us to think that she was an object for him (her beauty, for example, serving as a source of fixation for him for decades), the question of depriving her of himself was of the utmost importance, especially at the time that he told her that he would rather go live with his father than stay with her. His primary way of imagining having an impact on her was by hurting or harming himself—whether through drugs, illness, or suicide (driving off a bridge, for example). He would tell her about all kinds of stupid things that he did, trying to elicit expressions of concern and worry from her—indeed, he devoted a great deal of time and effort to finding ways to get her to worry about his physical and mental health. He often talked about his numerous physical symptoms—above all his myriad skin conditions—as messages to his mother and appeals to her for care and concern. (Recall that in hysteria, the repressed most often returns in the body.)

As a young child, he had once fallen off his bicycle and gotten several cuts on his face. When his mother saw him with blood on his face, she burst into tears. Harming himself was clearly a way to elicit sympathy from a woman, which he took to be a proof of her love for him, and he thought of his many skin diseases as unconscious attempts to elicit care from someone. (His father used to rub lotion on his back whenever he had a sunburn, and his mother put cream on his back at various points.)[17]

One might even speculate that an early scene in his life was a kind of critical moment as regards who was going to be able to secure the role of object *a* in the relationship between himself and his mother. After the parents' separation and eventual divorce, his father openly criticized his mother in front of J, and even went so far as to cruelly try to convince him that his mother was a bad mother and didn't love him (only his father did). One day when J was at his mother's house (before the divorce), being tucked into bed, he uttered a couple of words as though he were a baby, calling her "caca mama." This had a huge impact on her, for she apparently told him that if he didn't repeat what he had just said, she was going to jump out the window—the open window that she was standing next to, which was several stories above the pavement below. It seemed that she was perhaps not entirely sure what he had said and wanted to see if he had the guts to repeat it, but he told me that he was uncertain whether she was more likely to jump out the window if he did repeat it or if he didn't repeat it. She seemed to be putting herself in the position of the precious object that was about to be lost if he did the wrong thing, and in some sense we might say that there was a kind of battle or power struggle going on over who was going to be the precious object.

In the end, J said nothing. One could, in theory, deduce that to say nothing was to let her jump out the window, dare her to jump out the window, or even force her to jump out the window if she was going to be true to her word. In a sense, he might have been saying, "You are not the precious object, for I can allow myself to lose you—you are not essential to me. I am the one who is essential to you—you could never stand to lose me, for you would be devastated." The whole scene made a huge impression on J, and we might well imagine that it was a rather scary, high-stakes scene for a young child. But it could potentially be understood as the decisive moment in a kind of standoff or struggle between the two of them as to who was going to occupy the position of the precious object that the other cannot bear to lose: object a. If we accept this characterization of things, we again end up with the same formula for hysteria that we saw earlier: ($a \lozenge \bcancel{A}$). A precious object can be one that is especially loved or especially hated, as long as there is plenty of passion attached to it; J was a precious object that was, as he tells the story, primarily loved in the case of his mother, and mostly hated in the case of his father.

As I said earlier, J has a number of obsessional traits which can easily confuse the diagnostic picture, many of which grow out of his numerous identifications with his father. Although I have not been able to locate any particular way in which one could say that J was forcibly separated from his mother by his father, it might be hypothesized that J identified with his father as a way of putting some space between himself and his mother, having clearly felt smothered to some degree at home (recall that he slept in the same bed as her until he left to go live with his father). He described the very intimate moments where he and his mother would each tell each other how much they loved each other as suffocating in some way. After his father's death, some of that sense of suffocation returned, and he would even feel that his mother was somehow expecting him to "make a move on her," that is, make some kind of sexual overture to her, whenever they were visiting each other.

Apart from the kind of common identification with the father that we see in many young boys—for example, wanting to shave like his father did—J seems to have identified with the father's sense of having been unjustly, unfairly rejected by the mother, and yet being stuck on her for many years thereafter. Starting at around the age of nineteen, J would enact the same scenario again and again with his girlfriends: he would find a girl who was extremely interested in him, get her to fall in love with him, and then act like a monster to get her to break it off with him; he would sometimes do so by pretending that he had cheated on her when he hadn't, or by repeatedly insisting she didn't love him and making a big scene about it. As soon as she broke it off with him, he would become desperate and do everything possible to convince her to get back together with him. This was exactly what his father had tried to do with his mother for many years after they separated.

J's father was a monster toward his wife insofar as, when he was drinking heavily, he would come home and yell and scream at her. J himself was not much of a drinker compared to his father, but found his own ways to make himself unpleasant and annoying to his girlfriends, treating them like dirt, until they would finally get fed up to the point of breaking up with him. He at first thought of this as an attempt to test each girlfriend to see if, unlike his mother, she would continue to love and fully accept him despite his being a monster or being ill. His mother had viewed alcoholism as a disease, and he himself very quickly latched on to the idea that he had a disease as well: depression. With girlfriends he would oscillate between acting depressed and throwing fits of anger, effectively chasing them away just as his father had chased his mother away. The better looking the girlfriend was, the more he engaged in this repetitive behavior—recall that he considered his own mother to be a serious beauty and kept pictures of her from when she was around seventeen on display in his apartment and later on his phone for many years.

Early on in the analysis, he viewed it as part and parcel of his fate to be rejected by the woman he loved, a fate obviously modeled on his father's fate. Having learned as a child that his father had experienced a fairly long period of impotence after the divorce, J too became quite impotent with women after breaking up with the first really serious girlfriend he had in college, and that impotence has persisted to a greater or lesser extent for over two decades now.

An additional element of identification with his father concerns his physical health: his father had high blood pressure, and J has sometimes worried and he even almost had panic attacks about the idea that his blood pressure is off the charts (he imagined it being in the thousands instead of the hundreds!) and that he will die of a heart attack, his father having had high blood pressure and several heart attacks before he ultimately succumbed. His father took pills for his heart condition for many years, and J found a way to get himself prescribed all kinds of pills as if to prove that he was just as sick as his father was; indeed, by the time of the father's third heart attack, J was taking as many pills as his father was.[18]

J avoided going to see his GP for years at a time, saying that he was sure his doctor would tell him his blood pressure was through the roof.

He took the almost constant redness of his face as proof that his blood pressure was extremely high. So not only was he fated to live and be unloved like his father, he was also fated to die like him. Encouraging such intense identifications was undoubtedly the fact that they had the exact same first, middle, and last names. Indeed, J was rather taken aback at his father's funeral when the priest kept repeating the deceased's name, J getting the impression that he himself was being talked about as though he were dead!

Alongside these identifications with his father that we can situate in the symbolic register, however, we find a positioning of himself at the level of jouissance in a stereotypically feminine position. J engaged in quite a lot of early sexual play with (at least four) boys who were more or less his own age at the time (starting at age five or six), and virtually always occupied the passive, submissive, or bottom position with them. Most of these boys seemed more knowledgeable about sex than he was, and some of them were bigger, stronger, or more sexually mature than he was. He allowed them to do more or less whatever they wanted with him, only occasionally attempting to reverse the roles and become the active partner himself—often to no avail as his partner was not willing to go along with it. These early childhood sexual experiences with males seemed consonant with his later characterization of himself as his father's bitch for sleeping in the same bed as his father in the exact spot that his mother used to sleep. As he once put it, "To be dominated is to be loved."

These sexual encounters, in which he played the passive or submissive role, led him to wonder for years in the analysis whether he was not in fact gay. He would often worry that homosexual men wanted to anally penetrate him, such worry likely reflecting a wish on his part that they would want to do so. His father would often refer to him as a lazy good for nothing, because of his failure to study or work at things, but the expression that the father used included a slang term akin to "faggot" or "queer." Moreover, J felt that he derived too much enjoyment from defecating and from his anal zone in general.

All of this, combined with his feelings about being a coward, not standing up to bullies (or to his father like one of his friends had with his own father), made him wonder at times whether he was a man or a woman, although the form in which he sometimes raised this question was "Am I a master or a slave?" Some of the sexual activities he engaged in with certain girlfriends—for example, having them sit on his face and almost suffocate him—also made him wonder about this, as did the fact that at age nine he once tried on girl's clothing and makeup, and even to this day applies all kinds of creams to his skin to combat aging, the kind many women apply. Early on in the analysis, when I would ask him if we could change the date or time of a particular session, he said that he felt like I was breaking dates with him as though he were a girl, and that he would want to refuse in order "to play hard to get." For years when he was talking about a situation in which he was with a woman, he would say he was with "another woman." At one level, this could be understood to suggest that his mother was always implicitly present to mind as the first woman, but at another level that he himself was the first woman in relation to whom the second woman could be referred to as "another woman."

A certain kind of confirmation of his position as a woman, and not a man, and as object a can be found in one of his names. I obviously cannot reveal that here, for reasons of confidentiality, but the patient himself indicated to me that the name derives from a verb that means "to look." This does not make him the gaze itself, but it certainly is suggestive. In his flirting or dating activity, he almost never approaches a woman unless she has first looked at him and indeed smiled at him several times; indeed, I don't believe he has ever approached a woman who has not first looked at him and given him some sort of signal of her interest. Furthermore, he has often commented that he feels that he is so handsome that every woman should be looking at him and interested in him—that he is, in effect, God's gift to women! As he once put it, "Women should be fighting over me." In his fantasies of being a famous musician, "all the girls die for" him. (He once went so far as to say, "I want every woman to love me and every man to hate me.") He would often look at himself rather than at his female partner during sex, as though he were in love with and/or turned on by himself. Furthermore, he once professed that he identifies with the women in the pornography videos he watches who are getting "speared" from behind.

Fundamental fantasy

This leads us to the question of what his fundamental fantasy might be. Whereas he consciously deplores infidelity, sluttiness, and a craving for sex in women in everyday life—wanting women to be willing to forgo all sexual satisfaction in order to prove their unconditional love for him—in his masturbation fantasies he gets off on their infidelity, sluttiness, and craving for sex (for example, he often imagines a girl having sex with two or more men at the same time). In these fantasies, he is often with a young girl who says she is his little whore, loves sex, and can't get enough of it. She doesn't care a whit whether the sex is reproductive or not, which is what religion would tell her it should be. All she cares about is enjoying herself.

Moreover, the girl in his masturbation fantasies is often characterized as his daughter, he being a dirty old man who is having sex with his own underage daughter. Now, insofar as he identifies with the girl who is "getting it," as it were, in the videos he sometimes watches while masturbating, we might hypothesize that the girl he fantasizes about is in some sense himself: he is imagining himself as his father's daughter who wants to be sexually dominated and satisfied by her father.

In other words, although he is consciously horrified by the idea of being his father's "bitch," we might hypothesize that this is precisely the way he positions himself in his fundamental fantasy. Fantasmatically, he sees himself as a young, desirable object that the father wishes to possess and enjoy—as do all other men—an object that, moreover, also enjoys being possessed and gotten off on in this way. Although J often thinks of himself in everyday life as a dirty old man, there is, it seems, a level at which he sees himself as the precious sexual object for a dirty old man like his father.

Like many other heterosexual and homosexual men I have worked with who seem fixated on sexual partners who, in current terms, would be considered "underage," legally speaking, J derives a great deal of tense, anxious satisfaction from looking at online videos of girls who are supposed to be over eighteen, but who certainly do not appear to him to be over eighteen. He is often worried that the authorities who police pornographic websites will catch him looking at illegal sites where the girls are underage and throw him in jail for being a pervert; this tension and this anxiety constitute, in and of themselves, a form of jouissance. But I would suggest that what is really going on here for J, and for many other heterosexuals and homosexuals who are fixated on such underage partners, is that he imagines *himself* being the underage partner for a so-called dirty old man like his father was, in his view, when he was growing up.

What made his father seem like a dirty old man to him? Starting when J was little, his father would comment on J's girlfriends and on other girls he knew. I mentioned above that J had concluded early in life that women wanted men's money, and once, as a young child, he took a 100 dollar bill out of his father's wallet in order to give it to a girl he had a crush on in elementary school. (His father got him to give the money back.) At some later date, when his father caught a glimpse of that same girl at J's school, he commented that J had good taste in girls. When J was a teenager, he was at the seaside with his father once, and his father commented on how cute and sexy one of J's classmates was, a female classmate of J's who was there on the beach in a bikini. J was rather perturbed by this at the time, even though she was not a girl that he himself was interested in. He seemed disturbed by the idea that his father could be interested in a fourteen or fifteen year old. To his mind, only dirty old men were interested in adolescents.

It thus seems to me legitimate to hypothesize here that in his fundamental fantasy, J sees himself as the adolescent whore who just wants to enjoy herself with every dirty old man around, and especially with her father.[19]

It should be kept in mind that this is a fantasy and that J obviously would not want it to be realized—that is, to be played out in real life. He would not want some Other to actually get off on him. A neurotic fundamental fantasy is something the neurotic unwittingly enjoys as a fantasy, even though he could not bear to have it realized. Unlike what we might find in the case of a true masochist, J did not crave the actual physical punishment. He preferred the tension and anxiety of imagining that someone wanted to punish or dominate him. Indeed, on the one occasion on which the angry boyfriend of a girl he had slept with actually did punish him physically, he was clearly traumatized—it was something that marked him deeply and that he returned to repeatedly in analysis. In other words, like the hysteric, J wishes to bring out desire (e.g., to punish) in the Other but does not want to be the real object that brings the Other jouissance.

Now, if he would not actually enjoy being possessed and dominated by the Other, why would he have such a fantasy? If we think of J as a hysteric, the answer is perhaps quite simple: if J plays the part of a whore in relation to his father, this perhaps would, in his eyes, make his father into a real man—a strong, dominating man who was not impotent. This fantasy would thus be J's way of propping up a father whom he perceived to be weak in many ways. It would allow him to maintain a certain illusion, and help him prop up a strong castrating figure whom J would like to believe wanted to separate him from his mother. In other words, it would serve to reinforce or prop up the Name-of-the-Father, which he obviously considered to be somewhat lacking in power.

What, then, would it mean to traverse such a fantasy? It would not, I think, mean to come to be in the place of the dirty old man—which is, in fact, where he already sees himself in everyday life. Rather, it would mean to stop positioning himself as a whore for every Other with a capital O, for every male who comes along that he thinks of as a real man, as some sort of authority figure. It would imply no longer seeing himself as the cause of the misery or jouissance of all such Others, leading them to want to punish or get off on him.

How he would situate himself instead, I obviously cannot know in advance, but probably it would not be as a "real man" or "authority figure" himself. The further work of the analysis will presumably call into question for him the very notion of "real men" and authority figures. Were things to go further still, J would come to situate himself as the cause of his own desire—but we would have to wonder, then, his own desire for what? That remains to be seen.

Unconscious

In the course of this case presentation, I have mentioned quite a few ideas and wishes that we could understand to be—or at least to have been—unconscious for J (e.g., his skin problems as messages to the Other, his seeing himself as a whorish daughter for his father). Let me add just a few points here, by way of conclusion.

J clearly liked to think of himself as well accomplished, highly intelligent, and in no way lacking. Everyone else was lacking, everyone else was missing something, everyone else needed or wanted something from him, everyone else was castrated. And the more he secretly felt inadequate and lacking in almost all regards, the more desperately he tried to convince himself and others that he was not, going so far as to almost believe his own stories and fabrications (regarding his own history, his musical talents, his intellectual accomplishments, and so on).

He obviously saw himself as a kind of linchpin or link between his mother and his father (as we often see in hysteria), each of them trying to win him over to their side, each of them wanting him—or at least wanting to pull him away from the other parent. It would not, I think, be too much of a stretch to hypothesize that he wanted to believe himself to have been the cause of his parents' misery and ultimate divorce: he seemed to wish to believe that his mother loved him far more than she loved his father and that she perhaps divorced the father in order to be exclusively with her only child.

Undermining this wishful belief was the knowledge that his mother truly did love his father: she told him stories about seeing the father for the first time at a party and immediately telling her cousin that he was the one for her; and she howled in what appeared to be genuine agony and grief when J announced to her, almost twenty-five years after the divorce, that his father had died (J was the one who broke the news to her). The mother and father had remained in somewhat close contact for most of those twenty-five years, and had perhaps even had a brief dalliance or two when J was in his mid- to late teens.

This ignoring of what he knew again suggests what Lacan refers to as "moral cowardice, which in the final analysis can only be situated on the basis of thought—that is, on the basis of the duty to [...] find one's way around in the unconscious, in structure." The wish to be what one most profoundly senses one is not is perhaps always at the origin of the fundamental fantasy and leads to the most intractable misrecognition (*méconnaissance*).

Fantasy can be understood, as Lacan suggests, as the Other's desire. And since the Other's desire as such is unknown to us and can only be interpreted, fantasy can be understood as *an interpretation* of the Other's desire. J's fantasy can thus be seen as a wishful interpretation of his father's desire, an interpretation suggesting that it was J himself and not J's mother who was at the core of the father's desire; and that it was J himself and not J's father who was at the core of the mother's desire. I don't believe J ever consciously doubted that his father loved his mother more than he loved J. But he "worked hard," we might say, to get himself thoroughly enmeshed with his father. He strove to find a way to be at the center of his father's daily preoccupations. And J could at times delude himself into thinking that he, not his mother, was the most precious (albeit infuriating) object for his father.

* * *

Let me end today by indicating that, insofar as this is an ongoing case, nothing is yet fully set in stone, and I could be wrong about J's diagnosis and fundamental fantasy. I could obviously be wrong about these things even if the case had already come to a successful end. But insofar as it is far from complete, it is all the more important for me to remain open to hearing things that contradict or call into question my case formulation.

MIS-TRANSLATIONS

CHAPTER 8

What makes translating Lacan's work so difficult

(This paper was given in French at the University of Paris X, Nanterre, at a conference organized by the French Society of Traductology, held in memory of Umberto Eco, at the invitation of F. P. Alexandre Madonia, on June 6, 2017.)

Today I will outline three major difficulties facing all translators of Jacques Lacan's work, including both the work prepared for publication by Lacan himself and the work prepared for publication by others.

1. Problems with the "establishment" of the text—that is, of knowing exactly what the intended text is that needs to be translated.
2. Problems of comprehensibility of the text, including polyvalence, ambiguity, and, at times, apparent incoherence.
3. Problems of style, related to Lacan's different audiences at different times, and the style to be adopted by translators based on their intended audiences, whether their audience be primarily academic or clinical.

Although I will discuss these problems separately, they obviously overlap and intertwine.

Problems with the "establishment" of the text

I will begin with the problem of knowing what the text that we are to translate actually is. In the course of translating *Écrits*, I encountered hundreds of mistakes in the French text, which, regardless of who introduced them, were obviously left there despite the many reprintings of this major text by Lacan over the course of the last fifty plus years. In my translator's notes at the end of the book I signal dozens of errors and, in the main body of the text, I silently correct hundreds of others. Passages from texts written in Greek, Latin, German, and English are misquoted, proper names are misspelled, the texts cited are not always the ones Lacan was actually quoting from, and words are occasionally missing or misspelled to the point of unrecognizability.

One simple example is from the single-volume French edition of the *Écrits* (p. 470, paragraph 2), where we encounter *orinomante*, an apparent hapax legomenon, that is, a word found in no other text. After a great deal of research and consulting with several scholars, and intense study of the context in which it appears, I concluded that an inversion had occurred in the spelling of this word, which should read *oniromante*, referring thus to someone who reads the future, or engages in divination, by means of dreams (oneiromancy, from the Greek *oneiromantis*). We might be inclined to believe that Lacan was forging his own word, but he probably would have added some comment like *pour ainsi dire* or *si l'on peut dire* ("so to speak" or "as it were"), had he been doing so.

Despite the fact that the *Écrits* sold over 100,000 copies during Lacan's own lifetime, and has probably sold well over 200,000 in French in all, simple errors like this, which cause huge headaches to those who try to understand the text and indeed translate it, have—to the best my knowledge (I have not checked the latest reprinting)—never been corrected.

We can obviously wonder why. It seems that Lacan himself did not care terribly much about such things, being far more interested in what he was working on currently, and not what he had done in the past, in an ever-increasing race onward (*course ou fuite en avant*) to the next thing.[1] The translator is obliged, in such cases, to consult earlier-published versions of the individual articles collected in *Écrits*, which are often more accurate than their *Écrits* versions.

It would appear that, although François Wahl made valiant efforts to get Lacan to provide final versions of all of the texts that were slated to appear in *Écrits*, many errors were either left in or introduced into the texts by Lacan, by François Wahl, or simply by the typesetters and copyeditors. I provide a list below of some of the most obvious ones, which are of a rather wide variety of kinds, including some that are simply mistakes on Lacan's part, either owing to a misunderstanding of a text (especially in English), others that are typographical or grammatical mistakes (the first number corresponds to the page of the 1966 French edition, the second to the paragraph on that page):

> (13,4) Reading *trois* (three) for *dix-huit* (eighteen): Lacan seems to confuse the length of time he himself spent working on the combinatory analysis found in the "Suite" to "The Seminar on 'The Purloined Letter'"—eighteen months, as he tells us later (p. 39)—with the figure Poe provides when he has the Prefect say, "For three months a night has not passed …"
> (71,1) Reading *personne ne saurait* (no one knows) for *personne se saurait*.
> (132,1) Reading *faisaient* (plural for place) for *faisait*.
> (152,1) Reading *Je vous laisse juger de* (I'll let you be the judge of) instead of *Je vous laisse de juger*.
> (153,fn1) Reading "1946" for "1945."
> (160,4) Reading *C'est qu'il* (This is because it), as in the original version of the text, for *C'est qu'l* (obvious typographical error).
> (161,2) Reading *que partout ailleurs* (than anywhere else), as in the original version of the text, for *partout ailleurs* (leading to a nongrammatical phrase).
> (200,4) Reading *leur* (to the others), as in the original version of the text, instead of *lui* (to him).
> (335,2) Reading *un effet faux* (a false effect) for *en effet faux* (in fact false).
> (350,3) Reading *accordé à* (has in), as in the original version of the text, for *accordé*.
> (397,2) Reading *patrie* (homeland) for *partie* (part).
> (453,6) Reading *d'autant plus que* (all the more so since), as in the original version of the text, for *d'autant que plus*.
> (456,1) Reading *lit* (reads) instead of *dit* (says).
> (504,5) Reading *sache* (know), as in the original version of the text, instead of *cache* (hide).

(545,4) Reading *ailleurs* (as in the original version of the text, rendered here as "elsewhere") instead of *d'ailleurs* (moreover).

(628,7) Reading *un* (an), as in the original version of the text, instead of *en* (in).

(651,1) Reading *détonne* (stick out like a sore thumb) [...], meaning to be inharmonious or sing off key, instead of *détone* (detonate, explode, make a loud noise, or happen quickly).

(660,7) Reading *jaculatoire* (ejaculatory) instead of *joculatoire*, which seems to be nonexistent, although it may be related to the English "jocular."

(717,2) One might consider reading *suie* (soot), as in the original version of the article, instead of *suite* (pursuit).

(778,2) Reading *sadique* (sadist), as in the original version of the article, instead of *sadisme* (sadism).

(831,2) Reading *rassemble* (grouped together), as in the Desclée de Brouwer version of the text, for *ressemble*.

(833,1) Reading *beaucoup l'ont fait* (many have done so) for *beaucoup l'on fait* (meaning unclear).

(838,1) Reading *tenu* (said) for *stenu* (obvious typographical error).

(840,2) Reading *dans ce monde* (in this world) for *dans de monde* (meaning unclear).

Let me turn now to more general difficulties in establishing the text to be translated:

- Lacan often fails to cite his sources even in the psychoanalytic literature, or to cite them correctly or completely.
- He tends not to mention by name colleagues whom he is criticizing, such that the translator does not even know what texts to look at to figure out how to translate phrases or citations that Lacan has taken out of context.
- In his "Seminar on 'The Purloined Letter,'" he doesn't consistently put quote marks around phrases taken from Baudelaire's translation of Edgar Allan Poe's "The Purloined Letter" and rarely indicates when he is providing his own translation of Poe or is simply commenting on Poe's text.
- In his analysis of the work of Ernst Kris, his comprehension of the English text is so poor that it took him three tries—once in Seminar I,

once in Seminar III, and a third try in *Écrits* to finally grasp in which session Kris's patient said what and after which session Lacan believes that he acted out.

- In Seminar VI, his renderings of Shakespeare's *Hamlet* often leave much to be desired, and in the recent print edition of the seminar in French, passages that Lacan is quoting from Ernest Jones were obviously never consulted, giving the following text:

> *Un acte, c'est imparfait. Aussi peut-il donner au garçon le sentiment de la possession imparfaite de son propre pénis.*

Which might be rendered:

> An act is imperfect. It can thus give a boy the feeling that he imperfectly possesses his own penis.

But what we find in Ernest Jones's text is the following:

> Why should imperfect access to the nipple give a boy the sense of imperfect possession of his own penis?

The latter is obviously a horse of a different color!

It is, of course, quite possible that the stenographer misheard and/or mis-transcribed what Lacan said—Lacan perhaps read the text aloud in English, and native English speakers who heard Lacan speak English have unanimously reported that his accent was atrocious—but it is clear that in the process of "establishing" the text, Jones's article was never actually consulted. This seems hard to fathom, especially given the fact that for once Lacan explicitly references it.

As I have now crossed over into discussing texts that were published after Lacan's death, let me continue to provide examples from a seminar that I recently translated, *Seminar VI: Desire and Its Interpretation*. It must be a nightmare and something of a thankless task to try to establish a mostly faithful and accurate text of the seminars given the many homonyms in French, and if nothing else, the endless instances of the word *autre* (other) as a noun, which must be either capitalized or left lower case.

On pages 227–228 of the French edition of that Seminar (all page numbers given here from that Seminar correspond to the French edition;

they can be found in the margins of the English edition), where Lacan is commenting on a dream told by a patient of Ella Sharpe's, we find the following in the text regarding some of the patient's associations to the dream:

> *Le sujet est dans une voiture, il craint qu'elle ne tombe en panne, mais par cette panne, si elle se produit, il est bien loin de séparer qui que ce soit. Il arrête la circulation, il arrête sans aucun doute les autres, il arrête tout—nous le savons bien lequel est dans une voiture, bel et bien dans une seule voiture, qui les enveloppe tous les deux, comme la capote de la voiture qu'il évoque dans ses associations comme reproduisant le caractère de couverture de la caverne.*

Which translates more or less as follows:

> The patient is in a car, he is afraid it will break down, but with this breakdown, if it occurs, he is far from separating anyone at all. He blocks traffic, he undoubtedly blocks others, he blocks everything—this we know which is in a car, clearly in one single car, which envelops them, like the hood of the car he mentions in his associations as reproducing the character of the cave's cover.

The French text here is obviously incoherent, and if we fail to consult the original stenography and other versions of the seminar, we will be quite at a loss to translate it in virtually any way whatsoever, even if it is easy to guess from the context that there must have been something here about the King and the Queen insofar as they represent the parents in the patient's fantasy.

Other versions provide the following:

> *Le sujet est dans une voiture et, bien loin que lors de cet arrêt il sépare qui que ce soit, il arrête sans aucun doute les autres…*
>
> *qu'il arrête tout, nous le savons bien puisqu'il s'agit de cela, il est en analyse pour cela*
>
> *…tout s'arrête, il arrête [les autres,] le couple royal, parental, à l'occasion dans une voiture, et bel et bien dans une seule voiture qui les enveloppe comme la capote de sa voiture, celle qu'il évoque par ses associations, reproduisant le caractère de couverture de la caverne.*

Thus the middle part of the French passage would perhaps be better rendered as:

> He blocks traffic, he undoubtedly blocks others, he blocks everything—this we know because that is what is at stake, that is why he is in analysis—everything stops, he stops the royal, parental couple, which is together in one car, a car that envelops them ...

How are such errors possible, given the wide availability of the stenography and other versions of the text, both online and in libraries, and given the number of copyeditors and editorial assistants and colleagues who presumably read over the text before it went to press? One wonders.

Concerning this passage I added the following note at the end of the volume: "As a certain amount of text is obviously missing in this sentence, I have followed the stenography." The French editor subsequently demanded that all of my endnotes be deleted from the volume. They are available, however, on my personal website (brucefink.com) in the form of a pdf.

Many passages in the seminars suffer from the fact that the texts to which Lacan was referring were not consulted. For example, on pages 543–544 of Seminar VI, we find the following commentary:

> *Bref, il y a là toute une décomposition-recomposition, à quoi M. Gillespie rapporte ce qu'il appelle l'angoisse de castration. Dans le déroulement, interviennent aussi bien la primitive exigence, ou le primitif regret, de la mère, que l'identification de l'organe génital féminin à une fente.*

It seems to me that the French reader cannot have the slightest idea what "exigency" or "regret" is involved here, and Lacan perhaps abbreviated his remarks so much that this remained quite cryptic. When we read the text by Gillespie that Lacan is referring to we immediately learn that the patient's mother wanted him to be a girl and bitterly regretted the fact that he was not a girl. We also realize that the word "slit," which corresponds to the French term *fente*, is found nowhere in Gillespie's work, Gillespie talking constantly instead about a split or splitting, in other words, a *refente*. Gillespie rather bizarrely associates the splitting of the ego (Freud's *Ichspaltung*) with the fact that the female sexual organ appears to be "split in two," as he puts it, and he believes that the splitting of the ego for each subject stems from the image that the child sees of his mother's or sister's sexual organs.

Here is the translation that I propose:

> In short, there is a whole decomposition/recomposition that goes on here, Gillespie relating it to what he calls castration anxiety, including his mother's demand [that he be a girl] or regret [that he wasn't], and identification with the female genitalia as split.

In the notes I provide on my website, I add the following:

> The French here is very unclear in all versions, and the grammar is less than adequate. I have done my best to follow Gillespie's case study.

I add an additional note at the point in the French text where we see the word *fente* instead of *refente*:

> Reading *refente* (split) instead of *fente* (slit), the word "slit" appearing nowhere in Gillespie's writings, to the best of my knowledge.

In Seminar VI there are also obvious problems with the transcription of German terms, where in all versions of the seminar, instead of the fairly obviously intended term *Angst*, *Ansäße* (or *Ansässe*) and *Ansätz* or *Ansätze*, are provided (p. 137), none of which make any sense in the context according to my colleagues who are native German speakers, including Rolf Flor. I am not a scholar of German, but I can use a dictionary (even if they are not always reliable), and the German terms provided in the French edition do not seem to make any sense here. That edition could obviously have included the guesses made by the stenographer and those who were present at the seminar at the time, while indicating in a note at the back of the volume that these are mere guesses; but it doesn't.

In Seminar VI, *Schlagfantasie* is given instead of *Schlagephantasie*, as in the text by Freud that Lacan was referring to at that point (p. 151). *Rück-Phantasie* is given (it should at least be spelled *Rückphantasie*) when the context rather clearly requires *Zurückphantasieren* (p. 524), since Lacan explains the German term by saying *fantasme mais en arrière*, something which in English we call a "retrospective fantasy." *Hiflosigkeit* is given several times instead of *Hilflosigkeit*. And so on and so forth.

Lacan also occasionally makes slips of the tongue, which lead him, for example, to refer to "desire and the reality principle" instead of "the pleasure principle and the reality principle" (p. 140). Such slips are neither pointed out nor corrected in the French edition.

When I translated Seminar VIII, I had a terrible time locating quite a number of the passages quoted from Plato's *Symposium*, it seeming apparent that the Greek included in the seminar had not been adequately checked.

I realize that I am dwelling here on what perhaps amounts to perhaps no more than one percent of the overall text of each Seminar, instead of on the ninety-nine percent of what is well done, but it is that one percent that poses the greatest problems to readers and translators alike ...

Problems of comprehensibility

These problems regarding the actual text to be translated obviously also give rise to problems of comprehension. A great deal has been said about the incomprehensibility of Lacan's writing, so I will not broach that most generally, but only insofar as it poses problems for the translator.

First, no one translator can possibly catch all of the allusions to different people's work that Lacan makes, so I was led to consult with many other people regarding languages I don't know, specialized vocabularies, and references as I prepared the translation; but I have also been relying on the readers of the translation to help me improve it even after publication. Thus far I have received dozens of corrections from different sources, and have managed to get the publisher, W. W. Norton & Co., to make those corrections starting in the fourth printing. They have, however, stonewalled me as regards anything more substantive than changing a word or two here or there, so I have posted a list of additional endnotes on my website, along with lengthier corrections that the publisher will not allow. The translation thus remains a work in progress.

Second, translators have to grapple with how to deal with polyvalence and ambiguity in his work, for many sentences and passages allow for two, three, and sometimes even more different readings. The solution I adopted in *Écrits* is to provide in the main body of the text the reading that seemed to me to make the most sense at the time and given the context, and to provide alternative readings in the notes I included at the end of the volume. Here are a few examples of that:

(622,3) The French at the end of the sentence, *un certain passage du sujet au sens du désir,* allows for a number of other possible readings: "a certain movement of the subject in terms of desire," "a certain movement of the subject toward the meaning of desire," "a certain movement of the subject in the direction of desire," "a certain shift by the subject in relation to desire," "a certain shift by the subject as regards her desire," and "a certain shift of the subject as desiring subject."

(627,9) Regarding the "it" that speaks in him: there are too many masculine nouns in this passage (need, being, love, and lure) to be absolutely sure which one Lacan has in mind, though "need" seems quite likely. In the next sentence, *à sa place* (in its place) could refer to being's place, need's place, nonbeing's place, or even desire in its place or desire where it is situated.

(629,4) The grammar of the second sentence allows of a different reading: "demand evokes the want-to-be in the following three figures: the nothing that constitutes the heritage of the demand for love, the hatred that goes so far as to negate the other's being, and the unspeakable in what is not known in its request."

(677,6) The whole sentence here is open to different readings, for *est capable de précipiter l'identification du Moi Idéal jusqu'à ce pouvoir de méchef* can be understood in several different ways, such as "can even bring about an identification, on the part of the ideal ego, with the feeble power of mischief."

(856,7) *Une autre qui en fait* (another that makes it): the *en* here is open to different readings, as it could refer to "reality," "the reality principle," or even "psychical reality."

Perhaps the most complicated note I provided was the following, and it concerns only one part of a much longer sentence:

(626,3) The French at the end of the paragraph, *qui va du désir de son amie faire l'échec de sa demande,* is quite vague, and could also be rendered as "makes use of her friend's desire to thwart her own demand." The only request (*demande*) in question thus far in Lacan's discussion seems to be the friend's request "to come dine at the patient's house," but in the next sentence Lacan characterizes the patient's phone calls to caterers in her dream as a request as well. The desire most recently mentioned is the husband's presumed desire for his wife's friend, but the way it is expressed it could also be understood as the friend's desire for the patient's husband. Thus the patient "thwarts her own request due to her friend's desire for the husband or her husband's desire for her friend." Thanks to her "hysterical identification" with her friend, however, by thwarting her own request she also thwarts her friend's request to dine at the patient's home. *Sa demande* can thus imply "her own request" as well as "her friend's request," just as *le désir de son amie* can imply "her husband's desire for her friend," "her friend's desire for her husband," and even "her own desire for her friend," for (as we shall see) her husband's desire becomes her own.

The ambiguity and polyvalence of Lacan's work will never be eradicated, as a certain quantum of it was presumably quite intentional—think, for example of Seminar XX, *Encore*! All translators can do—assuming they do not attempt to adopt a position of mastery, do not profess to be masters of understanding—is provide the French in brackets, offer different possible renditions, and let readers grapple with the ambiguity and polyvalence themselves. This allows us to preserve some of the text's "signifierness" (*signifiance*).

Problems of style

- Lacan has a predilection for proffering impenetrable introductions to his papers and wrote a strikingly cryptic preface to the *Écrits* as a whole (if you have never read the first two pages of the book, have a look at them—they are about as off-putting as any written document could possibly be).
- He bends prepositions for his own wicked purposes, using them in ways for which there are few if any precedents in French usage, making it incredibly difficult to know what he intends by them (*sous* in "Logical Time," *par* in "Instance of the Letter," *de* in "Subversion of the Subject," and *dans* in Seminar VI).

These are the sorts of things that highlight the relevance of the Latin etymology of the verb "to translate": to carry across. To decompose it in my own way, I would say that each translator has to carry a cross, has a certain cross to bear, and deals with it in his or her own way.

Under the heading of style, I would also include the question of the enjoyment or jouissance of the text. This was a special concern of mine in translating Lacan's work on feminine sexuality in Seminar XX, where it was clear that Lacan was having quite a good time speaking in his ever more punning and multilayered way to his audience of 700. I attempted to convey in the translation the ways in which Lacan was really enjoying himself at the seminar, really having a good time.

But let us note the ambiguity in the phrase "enjoyment of the text." Is the text somehow enjoying itself? If not, whose enjoyment is it, the author's or the reader's? Is man's enjoyment the other's enjoyment? Not necessarily, I think. When an analysand is clearly getting off on something in a session, the analyst isn't necessarily getting off in the same way—indeed, certain analysands especially enjoy making the analyst anxious. And Lacan, no doubt, at times enjoyed making his audience squirm!

In his writings, especially prior to around 1965, Lacan did not enjoy himself in the same way at all. He suggested on the first page of *Écrits* that the style of a talk or text depends upon the audience: the style is the man one addresses (p. 9).[2] This might account for some of the diversity of styles one finds in the many varied papers in *Écrits*, some of which were delivered at international psychoanalytic conferences, some to students in philosophy, some to students in literature, and so on. As his audience changed, Lacan's style of address changed; this is especially visible in the change in style of his seminars over the course of the three decades during which he gave them, his audience having evolved considerably over those years.

The audience plays a role not simply in the author's style, but also in the approach adopted by the translator. For we have to ask ourselves, who are we translating for? Who is the intended audience of the translation we are painstakingly preparing?

I resolved right from the outset to prepare a translation of *Écrits* that was addressed to a different audience than the first English translation of a small selection of the texts in *Écrits* had been addressed to, which was an audience of philosophers and literary critics who were used to reading extremely difficult theoretical texts and were at least somewhat familiar with both French and German; that translation came out in 1977. After some thirty years in which Lacan's work was isolated in a small corner of academia in the English-speaking world, I decided to take seriously Lacan's claim in *The Four Fundamental Concepts of Psychoanalysis*: "The goal of my teaching has always been, and remains, to train analysts" (Seminar XI, p. 230). ["*Le but de mon enseignement a été, et reste, de former des analystes*"; 1973, p. 209].

My goal was thus to make Lacan's work accessible to English-speaking analysts who were not necessarily masochistic or in love with difficulty for difficulty's sake, who were not very conversant in Continental philosophy, and who were certainly not familiar with all of French literature from François Rabelais to Raymond Queneau.

As a practicing psychoanalyst myself, and as someone who was cognizant of the "turn away from theory" that was occurring in American academia in the 1990s, after several decades in which all things French were highly prized and at times even fetishized, I decided to prepare a translation for an audience of clinicians—even if it would require far more effort on the part of those practitioners than required by many of the texts in the contemporary psychoanalytic literature.

My working hypothesis was as follows: clinicians can get a great deal out of Lacan's work if it is translated carefully and accurately, with precise reference to the psychoanalytic texts by Freud and others that Lacan constantly refers to, and if the sentences are unfolded in a manner that makes them more readable—especially in English in which a multiplication of clauses and sub-clauses is rarely considered to be a thing of beauty, much less a joy forever, as it is by some in French. I am not a master of grammatical origami and would have found it very challenging to imitate Lacan's phrasal origami.

I provided extensive notes at the end of the volume to indicate what texts Lacan was referring or alluding to, and I made a choice not to try to invent a horribly difficult style for Lacan in English, but rather to generate a text that remains conceptually difficult but not stylistically difficult. In any case, for the most part, Lacan's stylistic effects are not translatable into English; to give just one example, in which Lacan clearly enjoyed putting an obscure adjective somewhat far from the noun it qualifies in order to create a striking or poetic effect:

> *En d'autres termes, le désir a à s'affronter à la crainte qu'il ne se maintienne pas dans le temps sous sa forme actuelle, et que, artifex, il périsse, si je puis m'exprimer ainsi.* (Seminar VI, p. 127)

Artifex seems—assuming I now understand it correctly, thanks to Matthew Baldwin, a Latin specialist I know—to qualify desire here, and can thus probably be understood as skillfully made, artistic, artificial, or ingenious. The fear being discussed here thus appears to be that desire, since it is an artifice, no matter how well crafted, may not endure. To locate an adjective in such a place in an English sentence would, in my view, simply render it altogether incomprehensible, unless a note is added explaining what it means and what it qualifies.

Consider the following stylistic effect, which seems to me far easier to understand (Seminar VI, p. 529):

> Ce phallus qu'elle peut avoir, réel, il n'en reste pas moins qu'au départ, il s'est introduit dans sa dialectique, dans son évolution, comme un signifiant.

Here it is at least obvious that the adjective *réel* (real) refers to the noun *phallus*. But in English one cannot insert the adjective "real" five words after the noun without at least adding the words "that is" (hence: *The phallus that women can have, that is real*), which weighs the sentence down. I thus translated it as follows:

> The fact remains that at the outset, the real phallus that women can have enters into the dialectic and its unfolding as a signifier.

My wager that clinicians can get a great deal out of Lacan's work, if it is translated carefully and readably, seems to have paid off: the new English translation of *Écrits* that came out in 2006 has sold over 33,000 copies in seventeen years.[3] New translation, new audience.

Let me end here with a few brief words about Lacan's notorious writing style, which has often been characterized as Baroque, and is generally believed to be inimitable. To quickly describe what Lacan does to the French language, I can do no better than to cite the comments of a music critic, Philippe Beaussant, on the compositions for the viol or viola da gamba written by the French master Antoine Forqueray in the late seventeenth and early eighteenth centuries:

> Every measure, every phrase, poses a problem and demands that the interpreter outdo himself. Forqueray indubitably took the playing of the viol to its zenith. There is viol music that is more tender and delicate, more radiant and sensual, more expressive and plastic. But none gives one the impression like this does of pushing the instrument to its limits, none manifests the same mixture of savage grandeur, excitability, continual violence, control, and power. [...] Forqueray seems like a knight who is always on the verge of working his horse to death, but who knows his horse too well to

go quite that far. [...] Excess was at the very heart of Forqueray's nature, and one cannot have the fire that burned in him without risking burning slightly whatever one touches. (From the liner notes accompanying Jordi Savall's CD entitled *Forqueray, Pièces de viole*, 2002) [my translation]

As you can thus see, Lacan's style of composition is situated within a previously existing French tradition. I have not attempted to work English to death in my translation of Lacan's *Écrits*. Rather, I have striven to do what the performer Jordi Savall does for Forqueray's music: make it look easy. Although I am sure I have not succeeded as masterfully with Lacan as Savall has with Forqueray, I hope that I have managed to render a Lacan who still burns slightly whoever reads his writings.[4]

"Foolish undertaking" and/or "Thankless task"

Translation tends to be equated in status with the lowly task of copyediting by most publishing houses, university presses, and college departments. "There is," as John Dryden (1992) says, "so little praise and so small encouragement for so considerable a part of learning" (p. 22).

Our beloved authors can make the occasional mistake or say something we disagree with, but our working assumption must always be that what they say is not sheer nonsense. We check all available editions for emendations, errata, and corrections of typos when we suspect something is amiss, but resign ourselves to the hard work of confronting something beyond our ken once we have exhausted such possibilities.

Just as the analytic situation itself puts the analysand in the situation of the beloved and the analyst in the situation of the lover who must not ask to be loved in return—he pays attention to what the analysand says in a way no one else ever has before, seeking to grasp the individual logic that guides it—translating puts the translator into the position of the lover who loves the text without asking to be loved in return. This is obvious in the case of a dead author, but is true even in the case of a live one who usually cannot appreciate the subtlety of the rendition. Love's flip side, hatred, arises from the seemingly inordinate amount of effort required in both cases—analyzing and translating—to make the work move forward. In psychoanalysis, this is tempered by payment. In translation?

If, as Friedrich Schleiermacher (1992) claims, translation is a "foolish undertaking" and a "thankless task" (pp. 40 and 52), at least it is not an impossible profession like psychoanalysis. The three impossible professions mentioned by Freud—educating, governing, and psychoanalyzing—all involve more than one person in situations in which the varied levels of each subject's will and jouissance interact, collide, and wear against each other. Translators have it easier: we have no need (or even opportunity, in most cases) to bring about change in any other subject than ourselves. And even when other people express little praise for our work, we ourselves may remain well pleased with it.[5]

CHAPTER 9

Lacan in "translation"

(This paper was prepared for a class given in December 1998 at the Advanced Study Center of the International Institute at the University of Michigan at the invitation of Slavoj Žižek, and delivered as a keynote address, at the invitation of Kenneth Reinhard, at the meeting of the American Lacanian Link, sponsored by the UCLA Humanities Consortium, March 5–7, 1999.)

> It seems to me that translating from one language to another [...] is rather like looking at Flemish tapestries on the wrong side, because even though you can make out the figures, they're partially hidden behind this thread and that thread, and you can't ever see them as clearly and with all the detail you can find on the right side. [...] Not that I mean to say translation can't ever be worthwhile, because, after all, a man could occupy himself with worse and even less profitable things.
> —Cervantes, *Don Quijote*

So-called French theory is, I want to suggest, a hoax in the English-speaking world—not, as Alan Sokal and Jean Bricmont (1998) have suggested in *Fashionable Nonsense*, because the French themselves do not know what they are saying, but because we are surrounded by unreliable translations of French texts. Violence has been done to "French theory" in English, the proportions of which should shock people in many areas in the social sciences, cultural studies, comparative literature, and modern languages.

The study of Theory has, for some time now, been displacing the study of languages and literature in many universities, and the result is that many graduate students and professors profess to understand texts they cannot possibly understand because they have no mastery of the language in which the texts are written. Nevertheless, given the stress in graduate programs on being able to employ terms and ideas from multifarious authors—who write, above all, in French and German—in order to produce "one's own original work" (as opposed to something more modest, like useful in-depth readings of one or two authors, or even just one or two texts), few people have the time or leisure to get close to a language, much less to the idiosyncratic language peculiar to any one specific author.

The result, as I see it, is that a great many people working in the area of theory, who base their work on texts originally written in foreign languages, have very little idea what they are talking about. If one relies on the current English translations of such texts, one may well be doomed to go astray.

On the production of translations

Let me begin with an obvious point about the *production* of translations in the English-speaking world today. Presses tend to provide few if any funds at all for translations of theoretical works. Only the translation of literary works with the potential for wider distribution seems to attract serious funding. The rendering of legal, financial, and other technical or business-related documents is, of course, better paid, because "real money" is at stake. This automatically means that translators with some genuine expertise are more likely to be translating future best sellers or legal contracts than philosophical texts. Who ends up doing the ill-paid or unpaid work of translating theoretical texts? Graduate students, for the most part.

Having been a graduate student myself for a fair number of years, I know that few of them have the opportunity to spend extended periods of time—and I do not mean one or two years—in a country where the dominant language is the one they are translating out of (the "source language"). Anyone who has lived for five or ten years in another language knows that you cannot get a real feel for a language by reading texts and looking up words in a dictionary, and that you are not automatically qualified to translate theoretical texts just because you speak a language "fluently." Fluency is a myth. You can speak a language fluently knowing only a couple of thousand words and avoiding the constructions you do not really understand. But does that mean you have a firm grasp on what people are actually saying when they speak to you? When you watch television, read a newspaper, or attend a lecture? Probably not—those things require a great deal of work with a language, a vast knowledge of idioms, and a great deal of experience with how idiomatic expressions are used contextually to mean very different things at different times.

Furthermore, even "genuine fluency" has little to do with translation ability. It is often noted by parents of bilingual children that their children have no trouble formulating what they want to say in two different languages, but are perplexed if asked to translate a question or term from one language to the other. They can speak both languages but cannot build a bridge between them. Translating involves a specific kind of praxis.

Even translators who live in the foreign country whose language they translate out of into "their own" (the so-called target language) may not find it easy to build those bridges, their relationship to their mother tongue having changed too radically during a prolonged stay abroad. Their ability to write and even recognize good—or even just decent or ordinary—English prose may become compromised (I have seen this repeatedly).

The upshot is that few people in general, and even fewer graduate students or untenured faculty (due to the pressures on them to publish quickly and plentifully), are in a position to produce even reasonably accurate translations of theoretical texts. If so many translations seem so abstruse and the prose style seems so stilted, it does not necessarily mean the original was atrociously written. It is probably more often true—to give the author the benefit of the doubt—that the translator did not really grasp what was being said and translated more or less word for word. George Orwell's comment is perhaps apropos when it comes to translations (though not more generally when it comes to Lacan): "The great enemy of clear language is insincerity." Translators most often present the reading public with obscure grammatical constructions when they do not have the faintest idea what the source text is saying—those are the times when translators resort to word-for-word translations (I should know: I have been led to do so myself on occasion).

The majority of translators are paid so poorly for the jobs they do that they can ill afford to take the time to go back over the text again and again to improve the style and try to get a better handle on the meaning(s). Alternatively or simultaneously, such sloppiness could be attributed to a general decline in standards of scholarship and publication, and to a willingness on the part of editors to accept poor-quality work, instead of requiring their authors and translators to do a better job. (The editors themselves are, of course, subject to certain economic and academic pressures.)

The Lacanian Thing

Turning now from the prevailing economic and academic conditions under which translations are produced, let us turn to the translations themselves.

Given my background, I have obviously been led to make my claim about the widespread misunderstanding of French theory on the basis of my examination of the texts by Lacan that have thus far been translated into English. I will take up a number of what I consider to be very serious mistranslations by well-known and lesser-known translators of Lacan's work: in particular, Alan Sheridan, Jacqueline Rose, Jeffrey Mehlman, and James Swenson.

Before I examine in detail their many and varied mistranslations, let me address what certain people are likely to retort: that Lacan is an exceptionally difficult writer and that, if there are so many errors in the translations of his work, it must be Lacan's own fault.

There is some truth in that retort: Lacan is a devilishly difficult writer and his French is very tough even for the French. But my first claim will be that Lacan's translators have gotten even the very easy stuff wrong. I am not referring to the obscure expressions only used by Madelaine de Scudéry, the terms from set theory most people in the humanities would never encounter in their reading, or the complex reflexive formulations that leave the text open to multiple interpretations. I am talking about mistakes anyone who has taken French 101 should know better than to make.

Example 1: In Jacqueline Rose's translation of Lacan's 1951 "Presentation on Transference" (Lacan, 1982, p. 64), she renders *les méfaits* [...] *du* [...] *physicien* (1966, p. 217) as "errors [...] of the physician." Now, one of the first things you learn—or at least should learn—in studying languages is that there are such things as "false cognates" (words that look and perhaps even sound alike in two languages but have different meanings), and that you absolutely *must* look up every word you are not positively sure of—and even then, what makes you so sure? In current French usage, *physicien* means "physicist," not "physician"; it has not meant *médecin* ("medical doctor") for a couple of hundred years, and Lacan was not commenting in this context on Rabelais or Diderot, either of whom might have used it in that way. Moreover, *méfaits* does not mean "errors," but rather "misdeeds" or "crimes." Given that Lacan wrote this text in 1951, it seems quite obvious that he is talking about "the physicist's crimes" against humanity—namely, the atom bomb. The next time your family doctor makes an "error" like that, I would recommend you run the other way!

Example 2: Faced with the French words, *les supposés psychologiques* (Lacan, 1975b, p. 78)—which even a beginner can diagram as article, noun, and adjective, in typical French word order, and adequately translate as "the psychological presuppositions (or assumptions)"—Rose comes up with "supposed psychologicists" (Lacan, 1982, p. 154). Have you ever met a "psychologicist"? Neither *Webster's* nor the *Oxford English Dictionary* lists any such word. You would think things like that would raise a red flag, if only to the unfortunate copyeditor who read the text prior to its publication.

Since Alan Sheridan is the best known of Lacan's translators, let us look at some of the simple mistakes he makes. Sheridan tells us that *attiger*, meaning to exaggerate or go too far, means "to transplant" (Lacan, 1977, p. 150; cf. *Écrits*, p. 416).[1] An *homme de cabinet* (Lacan, 1966, p. 642) is, in his book, a medical practitioner, whereas in everyone else's it is a scholar (*cabinet* can, of course, be an office, but *homme de cabinet* is a fixed expression). He confuses *rosière* with *rosée*, and translates the former as "dew" (which is what the latter means) instead of "virgin" or "virtuous maiden," which is what *rosière* means (*Écrits*, p. 419). Like so many translators of French texts, Sheridan gets the word order wrong in compound words like *souvenir-écran* (1966, p. 518). Even when a hyphen is added to such terms, the noun still precedes the adjective, in typical French word order, and the obvious psychoanalytic term "screen-memory" must be preferred to Sheridan's curious "memory-screen."

In all fairness, I should take Lacan's other translators to task as well; so let us consider one from James Swenson's translation of "Kant with Sade" (Lacan, 1989a). In the course of his discussion, Lacan says *"Le plaisir donc, de la volonté là-bas rival qui stimule, n'est plus ici que ..."* (1966, p. 773), and Swenson translates *là-bas* as "down there" (Lacan, 1989a, p. 62), as if Lacan were referring to the genital region with this term that has no such known connotation in French. Instead, Lacan is juxtaposing *là-bas* with *ici*, and, in the context at hand, the former refers back to Kant's system in which the concept of the will (*volonté*) plays an important part, whereas *ici* refers to Sade's system in which the concept of pleasure plays a crucial role. I would propose translating it as follows: "Pleasure, a rival of the will in Kant's system that provides a stimulus, is thus in Sade's work no more than ..." Swenson was perhaps misled by the plethora of references in this part of the text to male impotence, but the opposition between *ici* and *là-bas* should have tipped him off. If *là-bas* could conceivably refer to the genital region (and that is a stretch), what then would *ici* refer to here?[2]

Continuing in the vein of fairness, let me indicate a couple of errors that crept into one of my own translations—that of "Science and Truth," published back in 1989. In *Écrits* we find the following passage:

> Après quoi *le principe de réalité* perd la discordance qui le marquerait dans Freud s'*il* devait, d'une juxtaposition de textes, se partager entre une notion de la réalité qui inclut la réalité psychique et une autre qui *en* fait le corrélat du système perception-conscience. (1966, p. 856, emphasis added)

Now in Fink's translation (1989b, p. 5) we find the following:

> The reality principle accordingly loses the discordance that supposedly characterizes it in Freud's work when, due to a juxtaposition of texts, it is split between a notion of reality that includes psychic reality and another that makes psychic reality the correlate of the perception-consciousness system.

Note, first of all, that *après quoi*, meaning "after which," has been mistakenly understood as *d'après quoi* or *selon quoi*, making it less clear that a certain discordance in the notion of the reality principle is, according to Lacan, overcome *after* Freud develops his second topography (id, ego, superego). Note, secondly, that the *en* toward the end of the sentence is perhaps more likely to refer back to *il* (it) and thus to "the reality principle" at the beginning of the sentence, than to "psychic reality." (I have italicized all three of them in the French to make it easier to follow the grammatical referrals.)[2]

Let us now consider page one of Jeffrey Mehlman's translation of Lacan's "Seminar on 'The Purloined Letter,'" published in the venerable *Yale French Studies*. Mehlman's text reads as follows:

> [I]t is in the realm of experience inaugurated by psychoanalysis that we may grasp along what imaginary lines the human organism, in the most intimate recesses of its being, manifests its capture in a *symbolic* dimension. (Lacan, 1972, p. 39)

To anyone who has read no more of Lacan's work than "The Mirror Stage" and "Aggressiveness in Psychoanalysis," the notion that the human organism is captured in the symbolic dimension should not sound terribly Lacanian. "Alienated in the symbolic"—now that sounds like Lacan. "Capture in the symbolic," though, does not; despite Lacan's many paradigm shifts, "capture" does not seem to be one of the terms that moves from the imaginary to the symbolic. Let us look at the French, where we notice right away that the word "capture" does not even appear.

> C'est […] dans l'expérience inaugurée par la psychanalyse qu'on peut saisir par quels biais de l'imaginaire vient à s'exercer, jusqu'au plus intime de l'organisme humain, cette prise du *symbolique* (Lacan, 1966, p. 11).

Notice that Mehlman has gotten a couple of clauses in the wrong order, perhaps because he failed to see that the subject of the verb *venir* is *cette prise du symbolique*. It is *la prise du symbolique qui vient à s'exercer* here. If we correct it we find, *not* that "we may grasp along what imaginary lines the human organism, in the most intimate recesses of its being, manifests its capture in a *symbolic* dimension," but rather "we can grasp by what oblique imaginary means the *symbolic* takes hold in even the deepest recesses of the human organism." (I have also changed a couple of other things: the French provides *prise*, meaning "hold" or "grip," not *capture*; and *biais* is closer to "means" than to "lines.")

Note that this "slight error" completely inverts the meaning of the sentence. And that what might seem like a minor detail *completely changes the theoretical point being made.*

Why am I saying this? Because it might be thought that Lacan's translators, though fumbling certain details, have, nevertheless, grasped the main outlines of his thought, the principal concepts and structures. But where would they have gotten a clear idea of those concepts and structures if not from the individual sentences and paragraphs that make up Lacan's work? And if they make the simplest of errors—by neglecting to use dictionaries and by not doing their homework by looking up terms or talking with native speakers about idiomatic expressions (or not knowing French well enough to even recognize an idiomatic expression when they see one—after all, no one could possibly know them all, just as no one ever fully "masters" a language)—how could we possibly think they would do better when it comes to the difficult material?

The examples I have given, of which I have already collected hundreds in retranslating certain of Lacan's texts, do not involve the fine points of Lacanian theory, where we often encounter complex negations, subjunctives, convoluted sentence structure, obscure references, terminology from many far-flung fields, and the like. Hopefully, I have at least raised your suspicions about the possibility that the translators could have gotten the easy parts wrong while getting the tough parts right.

Theory in translation

Let us take a look now at a slightly more complex formulation. Here is an example from "Subversion of the Subject": "Sur le fantasme ainsi posé, le graph inscrit que le désir se règle ..." (Lacan, 1966, p. 816). The standard French expression, *se régler sur quelque chose* (to model oneself on something or adapt to something), is broken up here in a way that makes it a bit difficult to see and Sheridan obviously overlooked it. His translation: "On to the phantasy presented in this way, the graph inscribes that desire governs itself ..." (Lacan, 1977, p. 314).[4] Since when did Lacan say that "desire governs itself"? Unfortunately, there must be some hapless commentator out there (down there?) who has quoted and elaborated on this misguided notion in print; his or her readers then mulled it over—"I wonder what Lacan meant when he said, 'desire governs itself'"—and scratched their heads until they came up with some farfetched theory about how desire can be understood to govern itself in Lacanian psychoanalysis. Whereas, if we recognize the ordinary idiomatic expression here, we will translate the French more or less as follows: "The graph shows that desire adjusts to fantasy as posited in this way ..."[5] Once again, this is not yet heady theory—it is a simple comment about the Graph of Desire.

To give you a feel for the kind of violence that is done to theory proper by this kind of inattentive translating, let us examine a couple of passages from "Direction of the Treatment." The passages come from Section V, "Desire Must Be Taken Literally," subsection 6. One of the first requirements of a translator of Lacan's work would seem to be familiarity with Freud's work, and failing that familiarity, the translator should at least follow up those references to Freud's texts that Lacan actually provides.

The first thing to note is that Sheridan neglected to reread *The Interpretation of Dreams*, which Lacan explicitly says he is commenting on here. Sheridan thus seems to have no idea where the dream recounted by the butcher's wife comes from—which explains a number of his mistakes. Here is the French:

> Car ce désir de notre spirituelle hystérique (c'est Freud qui la qualifie ainsi), je parle de son désir éveillé, de son désir de caviar, c'est un désir de femme comblée et qui justement ne veut pas l'être. Car son boucher de mari s'y entend pour mettre à l'endroit des satisfactions dont chacun a besoin, les points sur les i, et il ne mâche pas ses mots à un peintre qui lui fait du plat, Dieu sait dans quel obscur dessein, sur sa bobine intéressante [...]
>
> Voilà un homme dont une femme ne doit pas avoir à se plaindre [...]
>
> Mais voilà, elle ne veut pas être satisfaite sur ses seuls vrais besoins. Elle en veut d'autres gratuits, et pour être bien sûre qu'ils le sont, ne pas les satisfaire. (Lacan, 1966, p. 625)

Here is Sheridan's translation:

> For this desire of our witty hysteric (Freud's own description)— I mean her aroused desire, her desire for caviar—is the desire of a woman who has everything, and who rejects precisely that.

> For her butcher husband is adept at supplying the satisfactions that everyone needs, he dots the 'i's, and he does not mince his words to a painter who is chatting her up, God knows with what end in view, on the subject of her interesting face [...]
>
> There's a man a woman could have nothing to complain about [...]
>
> But there you are, she doesn't want to be satisfied only at the level of her real needs. She wants other, gratuitous needs, and to be sure that they are gratuitous they must be satisfied. (Lacan, 1977, p. 261)

Note first that Sheridan mistakenly translates *désir éveillé* by "aroused desire," whereas the context of dreams requires "waking desire" or "desire in the waking state." This may appear to be a minor point, but it figures her desire for caviar incorrectly: in calling it a "waking desire" Lacan is telling us that it is a conscious desire *not* an unconscious one, whereas "aroused desire" leads in a rather different direction. Indeed, an important facet of Lacan's several page discussion of the dream concerns the difference between her conscious desire and her unconscious desire.

Note secondly that Sheridan erroneously renders *lui* and *sa* as "her" instead of as "him" and "his," respectively, because he did not locate the dream; there he would have seen that the painter flatters the butcher, not the butcher's wife. Here Lacan's commentary on the dream, to any English reader who recalls or takes the time to read the dream, already seems patently nonsensical.

Note thirdly that Sheridan altogether misses the negation (a not uncommon occurrence in his rendition of the *Selection*) in the last sentence of the passage quoted. Lacan is trying to say that the hysteric creates gratuitous needs, and the way in which she ensures they are gratuitous is by *not* satisfying them. For were she to satisfy them, she might become convinced that they were vital, not gratuitous. This important theoretical point—elaborated a few pages further on as the hysteric's desire for an unsatisfied desire—is completely lost here.

Here is my proposed translation of the same passage:

> For the desire of our witty hysteric (Freud is the one who characterizes her as such)—I mean her waking desire, that is, her desire for caviar—is the desire of a woman who is fulfilled and yet does not

want to be [fulfilled]. For her butcher of a husband never neglects to dot the i's and cross the t's when it comes to providing her the kinds of satisfaction everyone needs; nor does he mince words with a painter who flatters him, God knows with what obscure intent, regarding his interesting mug [...]

Here's a man a woman should have nothing to complain about [...]

But there it is: she does not want to be satisfied regarding her true needs alone. She wants other needs that are gratuitous and, in order to be quite sure that they are gratuitous, not to satisfy them.

It should be clear from this example that this is not rocket science. It is relatively straightforward commentary on one of Freud's texts, and it represents some of Lacan's simplest writing. Which does not mean it is easy to fully grasp—a number of analysts have devoted considerable time to unpacking it.[6]

Let us turn to a rather more difficult passage two pages earlier in the same text, where Lacan has just told us that Freud anticipated Saussure by discovering linguistic structure "[i]n a signifying flow whose mystery lies in the fact that the subject doesn't even know where to pretend to be its organizer." He goes on as follows:

> Le faire s'y retrouver comme désirant, c'est à l'inverse de l'y faire se reconnaître comme sujet, car c'est comme en dérivation de la chaîne signifiante que court le ru du désir et le sujet doit profiter d'une voie de bretelle pour y attraper son propre *feed-back* (Lacan, 1966, p. 623).

Here is Sheridan's translation:

> To do so, to find oneself as the desirer is the opposite of getting oneself recognized as the subject of it, for it is as a derivation of the signifying chain that the channel of desire flows, and the subject must have the advantage of a cross-over in order to catch his own *feed-back*.

Some readers may be so used to formulations like this that they do not even think twice about them. That is a very bad sign, indeed! Lacan does not write like that—only his translators or imitators do. He provides difficult but usually very precise formulations that make sense within the context of his work.

First of all, Sheridan fails to realize that *le* at the beginning of the sentence (*Le faire s'y retrouver*) refers to "the subject" in the prior sentence ("the subject doesn't even know where to pretend to be its organizer"). *Le faire* here means to get the subject to do something; to do what? *S'y retrouver*, that is, "to find his way" or "to refind himself there" (in "the signifying flow" in the last sentence), *comme désirant*, that is, as desiring. The *le faire* returns a bit further on as *l'y faire*, meaning "to get him [to do something] there"—to do what? "to recognize himself as a subject." Sheridan, instead, provides "getting oneself recognized as the subject of it" (which would be *s'en faire reconnaître*, not *l'y faire se reconnaître*).

Lacan is saying that if the analyst brings the subject to refind himself in the signifying flow as desiring, it is the opposite of bringing him to recognize himself in that flow as a subject. Why? Because desiring has to do with metonymy and prolongs the subject's alienation, whereas being a subject has to do with metaphor (see "Metaphor of the Subject," *Écrits*, pp. 755–758) and brings transformation in its wake. In other words, these are two different projects in which the analyst could engage the analysand.

The second half of the sentence is trickier, requiring one to have read the note Lacan provides at the end of the article, which mentions that during the talk he gave on which the article in question was based ("Direction of the Treatment"), he presented his Graph of Desire (*Écrits*, p. 692). One might then realize that, in the context of the Graph, *dérivation* means "branch circuit," "branch line," or "spur." A *voie de bretelle* is part of a cloverleaf or highway interchange, known as a crossover, which once again evokes the vectors in the Graph of Desire. Note too that *ru* means "brook," not "channel"; and that *profiter*, at least when rendered into American English, is "to take advantage," not to "have the advantage."

Reconstructing the latter half of the sentence, we find that

> [T]he brook of desire runs as if along a branch line of the signifying chain [imagine one of the vectors branching off from the left-to-right horizontal arrow of the signifying chain in the Graph of Desire], and the subject must take advantage of a crossover in order to catch hold of his own feedback.

I will not unpack the whole sentence here, but I think it is at least visible in this retranslation that Lacan is contrasting (1) the metonymic movement of desire from left to right along the signifying chain with (2) the subject who, in order to come into being (or "catch hold of his own 'feedback'"), has to engage in a retrograde, metaphorical movement from A to s(A).

Let me emphasize again that this is by no means rocket science. Since Lacan does not tell us he is specifically referring to the Graph here, it may seem somewhat opaque, but as soon as one reads the end note of the text, one retroactively realizes (if one had not already) that this is a direct commentary on the Graph, and a rather precise one at that. I am not claiming that it becomes a snap to understand as soon as it is more carefully translated, but I think *the reader at least has a fighting chance*.

This passage is by no means Lacan at his most difficult. But I think it drives home the point that Lacanian theory often turns into gobbledygook in English translation.

The examples I have discussed here are not a few extreme examples taken out of context to deliberately exaggerate the extent of the damage. Would that it were so! The fact is that on virtually every page there are serious errors of comprehension, sometimes several in a single sentence. Apart from the more recent seminars translated in the late 1980s and the 1990s, I would submit that *none* of the previously translated texts is reliable enough for gleaning even a passing understanding of Lacan's thought, much less for serious academic or psychoanalytic commentary.

Now for what I personally consider to be the icing on the cake: Malcolm Bowie provided us with an assessment of Sheridan's translation in his 1991 book entitled *Lacan*, published by Harvard University Press. To give you the proper background information, I should say that Bowie held a chair of French literature, was a fellow at that eminent institution, Oxford University, and wrote an earlier book, *Freud, Proust and Lacan* (1987), published by Cambridge University Press, not to mention two other books on French literature (published by Cambridge and Clarendon), all of which presumably rely on an in-depth understanding of French texts. In other words, Bowie would seem to have all the necessary credentials to make a cogent and trustworthy pronouncement about Sheridan's translation of Lacan's work.

What does he say? He writes that, in quoting from *Écrits: A Selection*, he has occasionally "modified Sheridan's generally excellent renderings" (Bowie, 1991, p. 214)! Who, then, was this Lacan his book was purportedly about?

My contention here is that translations such as *Écrits: A Selection* and *The Four Fundamental Concepts of Psychoanalysis* by Alan Sheridan, and *Feminine Sexuality* by Jacqueline Rose have done considerable violence to Lacan's texts and to his reputation in the English-speaking world. They are more than problematic: they are riddled with errors from cover to cover. Apart from a small number of analysts and critics, few have had the patience to sift through these incomprehensible translations to try to find the wheat hidden among the chaff. A few scintillating formulations have managed to get through into English more or less unscathed, and they have motivated many of us to further study Lacan's work, despite the obstacles posed by the texts we have had to work with.

It might seem foolhardy to so severely criticize the very texts that inspired me to move to France when I did in the early 1980s, but when one considers that Lacan is barely even on the map in American psychoanalytic and clinical circles, at least some of the blame must fall on the translations themselves. Yes, American analysts and psychologists may often be closed-minded and anti-theoretical, but there are a great many who have genuinely tried to read the major texts and thrown up their hands in despair. Bad translations—leading to vague commentaries on bad translations, giving rise in turn to still worse commentaries on vague commentaries—have done little to foster Lacan's reputation in the U.S. If it is as good as it is today, we have only Lacan himself and a very small number of his commentators to thank.

Sue the translator!

I mentioned earlier that I do not believe Lacan alone has suffered such violence at the hands of translators. I say that, first of all, because most of the translators I have taken to task here have produced other translations as well. Sheridan single-handedly translated five books by Michel Foucault (*Discipline and Punish, The Birth of the Clinic, The Archaeology of Knowledge, The Order of Things*, and *Mental Illness and Psychology*). Mehlman translated a variety of books by Sartre, Laplanche, Foucault, Blanchot, and others; James Swenson translated Balibar's *Masses, Classes, Ideas*; and Jacqueline Rose, while I know of no other translations she produced, wrote an influential thirty-page introduction to certain of Lacan's texts in *Feminine Sexuality* and has been instrumental in introducing French work on feminine sexuality into the English-speaking world (see her book, *Sexuality in the Field of Vision*, which includes discussions of Kristeva and Lacan)—on the basis, of course, of her "knowledge" of French.

Add to this the fact that many other prominent French authors have extensively quoted or referred to Lacan over the years, and that when their texts are translated—their translators usually drawing on Sheridan's and Rose's work—the mistakes are merely compounded. While I will not discuss in detail the translations of texts by authors other than Lacan here, I hope I have at least rendered plausible my thesis that some modicum of violence has been done to their work as well and thus to French theoretical work more generally.

I will leave it to the reader to imagine exactly what that means given the relative popularity of "French thought" in the English-speaking academy today. What exactly is it that has become so popular?

I frequently hear it said nowadays that "we" already know Lacan's work and have in fact gone beyond it—a statement I find as astonishing as Lacan found the title of a talk one of his colleagues gave, which was "Knowing Freud's Work Before Translating It." As Lacan indicates, such a title is positively preposterous, for we must obviously first work at translating Freud's work before we can in any way, shape, or form claim to know it: "To know Freud's work before translating it ineluctably implies the following stupidity: knowing it before having read it" (Seminar XIV, p. 214).

* * *

I will end this talk with a plea, a plea that those of you who are genuinely interested in studying Lacan and putting him to use in your various areas *learn French!* Not superficially, not a smattering here and there, but a total immersion, for as long as possible. If you are making a claim, in a class or in print, on the basis of the interpretation of a couple of crucial passages in one of Lacan's texts, you should make damn well sure your translator got it right. How do you do that? By doing your homework.

I would argue that there is an easy way to separate the good translators from the bad, and the good interpreters of Lacan's work from the bad: when your interpreter or translator says, "it's not French" or trots out the French cliché, *"c'est pas du Français, c'est du Lacan,"* run the other way. Because the more closely you research Lacan's language, the less invention you find—the more you find that Lacan is borrowing from Madame de Sévigné here, from Marguerite de Navarre there, and from as far-flung fields as pyrotechnics and network theory. *It is French*—it is just not your everyday, run-of-the-mill French. (Invention, of course, becomes rather more prominent in his work starting in the late 1960s.)

If your translator or interpreter says she "has the impression" that a certain expression might mean this or that (and I have heard this on many occasions), do not take it lying down. Demand that she show you *that French usage allows for such an interpretation!* Demand that she show you that the context, the author being alluded to, or the grammar of the sentence allows for such an interpretation. The "sliding of the signifier," a formulation that is often bandied about, was never intended to imply that Lacan's signifiers can be taken to mean anything and everything we want them to mean. In fact, this formulation is found only once in Lacan's work, to the best of my knowledge, and concerns the subject's slippage from one object of desire to another, not the impossibility of meaning: *un sujet soumis au glissement infini du signifiant*, "[subjects] subjected to the infinite sliding of the signifier" (Seminar VIII, p. 171). In the context in which Lacan utters these words, the idea is that object *a* puts a stop to the subject's sliding from one object of desire to another, for example, from one fungible partner to another. A formulation that we find more often is the "sliding of the signified under the signifier" (*Écrits*, pp. 419 and 425). This latter means that the signifier's meaning is not fixed once and for all; rather, it can change as the result of new metaphorical uses of the signifier and through the latter's metonymic associations with other signifiers.[7] When Lacan gives a signifier a new meaning, he usually makes this quite clear. Otherwise, his use of language is very much grounded in French usage—not always the most common French usage, but usage that is attested to, nevertheless, in French literature and theoretical texts.

My goal is to encourage readers to take Lacan's text like an analysand's discourse: before considering what it means, let us take a very long look at what he or she actually said. The worst abuses of analytic treatment arise when the analyst jumps to conclusions about what the patient means, instead of focusing above all on what he or she actually says. Arriving at a global conception of the meaning usually needs to be deferred for quite a while (and may not be of much use in the treatment, ultimately).

The same is true when reading Lacan: *the meaning is very often something other than the first meaning that comes to mind.* You may already be familiar with a word you come across in his writings, but you still have to look it up because it usually has other meanings too—medical, psychiatric, legal, or financial meanings of which you might not be aware. This involves going through the 22,000 pages of the *Trésor de la langue française* (which can, at least now, be consulted online) and a long bookshelf of other more specialized dictionaries as well. Which, for most of us, is not all that exciting; nevertheless, that is what is required to read Lacan.

I would like to propose that a translation be thought of as a contract of sorts: when you make a big mistake in translating, it is as if you had left a gaping loophole in your contract and someone winds up suing you. Currently there is no price to pay for translating incoherently in the academy in the United States and other parts of the English-speaking world. There should be!

In the world of professional translation, where people are paid substantial sums to translate legal, financial, and medical documents, translators pay a price for screwing up: they get fired. Why? Because the so-called end user—the reader—may wind up harming or killing someone if she follows incorrectly translated instructions, telling her to adjust some newfangled instrument to the wrong setting; and that reader may then go on to sue the manufacturer who hired the translator.

But when it comes to the translation of theoretical texts in the humanities, translators do one lousy translation and the press gives them more. Why? Because their editors and readers do not demand any better.

We should start holding publishers and their translators more accountable for what they produce. For what they produce has very real effects! Psychoanalysis is, at least in large part, a text-based praxis, a praxis that is transmitted through the study of texts. Many analysts look to translations of Freud's work for ideas about how and how not to practice; and some of them also look to the translation of Lacan's "Direction of the Treatment" to see what Lacan says about interpretation and where he claims the analyst must situate herself when she interprets.

Lacan introduces an intriguing metaphor for the analytic situation in "Direction of the Treatment," based on the game of bridge which involves four players. I will not go into the details here (as I have done so elsewhere),[8] but he tells us there that "the analyst strives to get the analysand to guess (*lui faire deviner*)" the fourth player's hand

(*Écrits*, p. 492), the fourth player being the analysand, not as ego, but as subject of the unconscious. Alan Sheridan had Lacan recommend to the analytic world that the analyst "try to expose" the fourth player's hand (Lacan, 1977, p. 229). Yet there is a whole world between recommending that *the analyst expose the analysand's hand* and that she, instead, *get the analysand to guess his own hand*, and that world is the world of mastery. It may be a short sentence, but it marks the giant step Lacan takes away from many analysts of the International Psychoanalytical Association who often see themselves as masters of knowledge, able and willing to expose the analysand's unconscious, ready and able, owing to their astounding "powers of insight," to pinpoint the subject's mainspring and reveal it to him. If the analyst is to get the analysand to guess his own hand, the analyst must be operating as object *a*, not as some sort of all-knowing subject.

Should we be surprised if more mastery-oriented therapeutic work grows out of such sloppy renderings? I say: *sue the translator!*[9]

MIS-SPEAKINGS

CHAPTER 10

The emphasis on the unconscious is back

(Interview conducted by Tobias Wessely and Pablo Lerner in Copenhagen on April 14, 2018. It appeared in *The Scandinavian Psychoanalytic Review*, *41*, 1 [2018]: 44–51.)

"Psychoanalysis is not a philosophy, it's a practice."

Tobias Wessely (TW): How did you become interested in psychoanalysis, and especially in the French tradition?

Bruce Fink (BF): I became interested in psychology very early on, during my teenage years. I was always trying to understand people, understand love, understand life. I encountered the work of R. D. Laing fairly early on, and around the age of seventeen I discovered Freud. I studied quite a bit of psychology during my undergraduate years at Cornell University, but I had other more political and philosophical aims at the time. In my early twenties, one of my friends talked to me about French theory and we sat in together on a class offered in the Department of Romance

Studies at Cornell on Foucault, Barthes, Derrida, Lévi-Strauss, and Lacan. That's how I started reading Lacan. I didn't understand much, naturally, but I was very intrigued by his notion of the subject and the way he talked about the unconscious, which I hadn't heard talked about in that way at all in America. I was unhappy with the U.S. for all kinds of reasons at the time and I thought, "Why not go to France for a year or two and see what this Lacan stuff is about?" I ended up staying for seven years and doing all of my analytic training there.

Lacan had just recently died when I arrived in France in 1982. I was lucky, because there was a huge proliferation of Lacanian groups at the time and a kind of a renaissance in Lacanian thinking. My sense was that in the last ten years of his life there was such reverence for the Master that few could think outside of his system. I went to different institutes and heard a lot of different people speak. I studied philosophy and attended classes with many interesting people, like Badiou, Derrida, Deleuze, and Guattari. I was like a kid in a candy shop, there were so many interesting things going on! And, most importantly, I went into analysis for personal reasons.

In the end, I decided to do my graduate studies in Paris. I hadn't planned to in advance. I went there at first to do my own analysis—having no idea how long it would last—and to study a bit, without realizing it would determine the course of my life.

TW: What kind of place does Lacan have in America today? Has it changed in any way over the years?

BF: It has changed, very much so. In the late 1970s and early 1980s, Lacan was known primarily to literary, art, and film critics. The situation was much the same when I returned to the U.S. in

1989, but I personally devoted the lion's share of my efforts to presenting Lacan clinically.

Now, thirty years later, Lacan is read by at least as many people in clinical fields as in other more strictly academic fields. I was really struck by something that occurred when I was translating Lacan's 900-page *Écrits* into English, which was a very long and difficult process, as you might imagine, taking me the better part of ten years. I applied to the National Endowment for the Humanities (NEH), a federal agency that supports cultural endeavors, for grant money. The first time I applied, I received quite a lot of money, which translated into a considerable amount of release time from teaching for two years at my university, allowing me to focus on the translation. When I applied for further grant money in 1999, the NEH sent my application out for review, as they usually do, to a variety of professors. One of the professors made the following comment: "I thought Lacan was *passé*." To his mind, Lacan was no longer trendy, no longer of any interest.

Fortunately, I managed to finish the translation anyway and it has now sold over 30,000 copies, considerably more than the older version which was read primarily by academics. My impression—and a lot of people tell me this is true—is that psychiatrists, psychoanalysts, and psychologists are now actually reading Lacan's work, which is new. There aren't many analysts in America who can help teach people a Lacanian clinical orientation, but more and more practitioners are reading his work nevertheless. My sense is that a lot of the young people in training at institutes in America feel they have reached a dead end somehow. They're not very interested in or convinced by what is being taught to them at their institutes and are looking for something else. Very often it is the analysts-in-training who ask their institutes to invite Lacanians to come give talks and classes.

Pablo Lerner (PL): What can Lacan, or Lacanian theory and practice, say or do about the American way of life?

BF: Well, the American way of life (laughs), that's a really big question! I'm not sure what impact it can have on the American way of life. I think at least it can help counter an engrained American way of thinking, namely that psychotherapy has to be streamlined and totally goal-oriented. Which is the way Americans think about a lot of things, including education, business, and politics! And it goes for psychotherapy as well, Americans being the ones who have introduced forms of therapy that are supposed to work after only six or maybe ten sessions. Lacan brings a breath of fresh air into that sort of approach. To him, psychoanalysis is a non-goal-oriented project. In most forms of psychotherapy today, the buzzword is "symptom relief" or "symptom removal," and you have to provide a quantitative read on such relief after every session. Lacan provides a very different way of thinking about symptoms, which are sometimes essential if people are to go on living in the world. I think Lacan can contribute a lot to changing the public's views of what psychotherapy should involve.

TW: Would you say that there is something Lacan has to offer that especially resonates with younger clinicians in America today?

BF: There are probably a number of things. Especially Lacan's emphasis on Freud, on actually reading Freud, and of course his emphasis on the unconscious. Up until about ten years ago, people didn't read Freud much anymore. What I hear now is that institutes are beginning to offer year-long and sometimes even two-year-long courses on Freud. So interestingly enough, Lacan seems to have sparked yet another return to Freud. The emphasis on the unconscious is also back. I think a lot of younger clinicians find the work that they are usually encouraged to do—which is all about the transference and the countertransference—exhausting and emotionally draining. I suspect that the Lacanian approach is less exhausting to them personally.

I receive a lot of invitations to speak at institutes and almost all of them come from the new generation of trainees. Some of the more established analysts come to my talks and some of them are a bit open, but in general it is the analysts-in-training who are most interested. Here's a silly example: I've been living in Pittsburgh for twenty-five years now, and I taught at Duquesne University for twenty years. The first year I was in Pittsburgh I made contact with the Pittsburgh Psychoanalytic Center, which is affiliated with the APA. They clearly wanted nothing to do with me. Twenty-three years later, once the older generation of analysts had either died, retired, or simply withdrawn from the main decision-making positions at the institute, I suddenly received a call asking me to come and teach a course on Lacan for them. "Who are you?" I had to ask, "Where did you come from (laughs)?" Now they ask me to teach a course on Lacan or Freud every year, whereas I was *persona non grata* for decades. So, it seems to me that there's a generational shift occurring.

I think a number of the younger people also have broader intellectual horizons and backgrounds than their teachers. Many of them come from philosophy, literature, or political theory, and they learned about French theory in college before deciding to study psychoanalysis. Which is nice, because there is a very strong anti-intellectual trend in America. Many older analysts focused almost exclusively on medicine right from the beginning of their studies and don't know a great deal about other fields. In contrast, a lot of younger analysts are interested in literature, art, music, and politics, which makes things a lot more fun!

PL: So there's a changing landscape in America where psychoanalysis—Freudian and Lacanian—can perhaps …

BF: … get its foot in the door, yes!

PL: Can you say something more about that, you not only being a psychoanalyst but also having worked as a university professor. How is Lacan received in psychology departments in the United States? Is he regarded as a serious thinker? Or is he just considered to be an outsider?

BF: I think he's still seen as an outsider. I left the university five years ago, never having been particularly fond of academic teaching for a variety of reasons, one of them being that psychoanalysis is rarely accepted in psychology departments. I was lucky because the department I was in had a philosophical orientation. Their roots were in "existential-phenomenology," as they called it, so they were somewhat familiar with French and German theory, Heidegger, Merleau-Ponty, and things like that. They hired me by mistake, as I always like to say, by accident: they thought Lacan was a phenomenologist! They had no idea he was a structuralist and didn't seem to realize he was a psychoanalyst.

Freud, to many of them, was *anathema*. Some in the department hated Freud with a passion. And it was only their misunderstanding of Lacan that allowed me to get a job. No other psychology department in America at the time would have hired me. I know that because I applied elsewhere repeatedly.

Up until the 1970s, many psychology departments did have one psychoanalyst on staff. A lot of psychiatry departments would also have one, maybe even two psychiatrists who were also psychoanalysts. Starting in the 1970s, however, the medical model became so dominant that the analysts were either fired or simply not replaced when they retired. And psychology departments never replaced their analysts who retired. There are almost no psychoanalysts in psychology departments in the United States today. There are a few exceptions, of course. A few former students of mine who are brave enough to indicate on their CVs that they are interested in psychoanalysis and Lacan have managed to get university jobs, but usually in very peculiar psychology departments that have historically had a philosophical orientation. There are probably five of them in the whole country. So it's not easy. In clinics in the United States, it's very difficult to be accepted if you are a Lacanian. Most people think you're some sort of strange being from another planet, so Lacanians tend to hide their interest in psychoanalysis when they apply for clinical positions. But little by little, things seem to be changing.

TW: So you can see this change among clinicians. Would you say that patients are looking for a Freudian or Lacanian analyst, or even for a psychoanalyst? Or are they just going to therapy?

BF: I would say that the majority are just going to therapy. But I think that one thing that is working in our favor is that Lacan has been read by a lot of people in the universities; he's read by a lot of people in philosophy and in political theory as well. Slavoj Žižek has kicked open the door to Lacan even in many undergraduate courses. I get contacted by a lot of younger people who want to do a Lacanian analysis. They don't really know anything about it or what it involves. But they've read some commentaries on Lacan that lead them to think he's a radical leftist—which is hardly true—and they'd rather do therapy with someone whom they presume to be on the left. Often they want to do something that is countercultural. Maybe their parents are willing to pay for them to go into therapy, but they're certainly not going to see the type of therapist the parents want them to go see.

Do people actively seek out Lacanians in Sweden?

TW: I wouldn't say so. They look for therapy, and by recommendation you get a name. I wouldn't say that many patients even know they are going into analytic therapy, really.

PL: There is a small group who, since Lacan has gotten almost a mythical status, think it's kind of cool to go into Lacanian psychoanalysis, and they of course seek Lacanian analysts. But the majority don't know what they're up to.

BF: That's true in the States too. It's a very small percentage, often a very highly educated group that already knows something about Lacan.

PL: Now that we're talking about the intellectual discourse where Lacanian psychoanalysis has in a way taken root, what do you, as a clinician who also has a place in this discourse, think the clinical dimension can do to affect or transform it? Sometimes you get the feeling that it's very detached from the experience Freud and Lacan are very close to, namely the clinical encounter. Can it contribute in any way?

BF: I hope so. It's funny because in a certain sense there's been a parallel phenomenon in the

United States, which is that both my own work and Slavoj Žižek's work have become very popular at the same time, usually in different audiences, but sometimes in the same audiences. It's hard to say how they have really influenced each other. As I said earlier, I think Slavoj has sparked a lot of people's interest in going into psychoanalysis for themselves. Some of them start out in philosophy departments; they get their undergraduate degree in philosophy, and then decide to go into psychology, because they want to become analysts. But I'm not sure how much clinical discourse has affected academic discussions thus far. I know some of my colleagues in philosophy read my books and other books on clinical issues. But I don't know what effect such reading has on their work and how they approach things. Maybe that remains to happen or to be seen.

TW: You said that you had political interests when you were younger. And there is a history of ties between critical theory, the left, and Marxists, on the one hand, and psychoanalysis on the other. What would you say is the relation between psychoanalysis and politics?

BF: I think it's very complex, but I don't think psychoanalysis lends itself to any one particular political platform. It helps us see the degree to which each political standpoint is a kind of ideology, and to look at each of them as a system that allows us to see certain things and blinds us to other things.

I know that there are a lot of Lacanians who want to analyze Donald Trump and they really go to town with it. Personally I don't think that's a very interesting thing to do, since Trump is not on their couches and they are thus analyzing "wildly," projecting a good deal. I think psychoanalysis can help us look at right-wing, middle-of-the-road, and left-wing politics, and think about what's at stake in each. And it can help us see the contradictions in each person and grasp why they adopt certain political opinions. At least at a personal level it allows each of us to ask ourselves some questions when we're on the couch: "What led me to adopt a certain political stance?" "What am I running toward?" "What am I running away from?" "What am I hiding from myself?" I think it gives us a lot of clarity about our own political positions.

I'm not someone who tries to apply psychoanalytic concepts to other realms than the clinical realm. Slavoj does that all the time, and perhaps owing to his influence there are a great many people who apply notions like the real, *jouissance*, and so on to political systems. I have my reservations about doing that. I think I understand why they're doing it, but I'm not convinced of the validity of doing so. My impression is that, in their usage, psychoanalysis becomes a kind of philosophical system. To me psychoanalysis is not a philosophy, it's a practice.[1]

PL: Do you think that Lacanian theory and practice can vitalize or de-ideologize Lacanian institutions?

BF: I would say yes, but I don't think it's happening. History seems to suggest that the people who are at the heads of many of the psychoanalytic institutes that profess to be Lacanian are incredible ideologues! Psychoanalysis should make people suspicious of their own motives. You would think that, since the analysts who work together in institutes have all gone through their own analyses, their initially grandiose sense of themselves would have become tempered, and that they would understand something about their own egos and unconsciouses—which would, in theory, allow psychoanalytic institutions to function better than other institutions. But they don't. Analysts at institutes fight like cats and dogs for power among themselves. Let me give you just one example. In Pittsburgh there were at one point three Jungian psychoanalysts working together, and they had to split into two different groups because they just couldn't get along. The same is true for Freudian analysts, Lacanian analysts, and so on. You would think that a genuinely psychoanalytic institute that really applied psychoanalytic concepts might allow people to find a way to get along and really discuss things, share power, and so on. But it doesn't seem to be the case.

TW: Is there any exchange of ideas, any ongoing conversation between different perspectives, different schools in America? Perhaps not between institutes, but between people?

BF: Always between individuals: there are often friendships that develop between people from different schools. There are also certain institutes, like NPAP in New York, that are more eclectic. At NPAP, you can take a whole course on Lacan, Freud, Bion, or Klein. Nevertheless, training programs generally have a specific overriding orientation, but they're opening up a little bit more. What's happened essentially in the United States is that the old IPA-affiliated institutes almost died at a certain point, about twenty to twenty-five years ago. There were almost no new candidates. Nobody wanted to study psychoanalysis anymore at those places. But the newer institutes that were either Jungian or Kleinian or relational began to grow. Those are often the most vibrant ones now. The older institutes are trying to open up more, little by little, but they're often struggling.

Maybe someday there will be more Lacanian institutes. There are two small ones right now, and a couple of others that are perhaps in the process of being created.

PL: What do you think about the future, the place of Lacanian psychoanalytic theory and practice in the United States?

BF: I don't spend much time trying to predict the future. I hope the trend will continue. To my mind, it's only worth continuing as long as the Lacanians are serious ones and not charlatans. Unfortunately, as in any country, in the United States we had, early on, a certain number of people who called themselves Lacanians who were terrible theorists, horrible practitioners, and really gave Lacan a bad name. If it's quality work that they're doing—great! If not, let them stay at home, let them go somewhere else. I think that's true everywhere: in France and South America, for example, Lacan became incredibly popular, but only a small percentage of the people who call themselves Lacanian are doing credible work.

TW: What would you say are the main challenges for psychoanalysis today in American culture?

BF: In American culture, and in French culture as well, the biggest challenge is the medical model of psychiatry, which maintains that every problem is due to a chemical imbalance in your brain which can best be treated with drugs. The other main challenge is cognitive-behavioral therapy and other very short-term goal-oriented therapies. As you may know, most people in the U.S. have private insurance, and private insurance almost never pays for psychoanalysis. In fact, it rarely even pays for long-term psychotherapy; at most it may cover once a week sessions for thirty weeks. If a psychologist wants to see someone for more than ten sessions, he or she may have to give the insurance company a diagnosis which could potentially be damaging to the person later in life, because it stays on records which could someday become public. So we have to deal with the medical model and the insurance model, and then there is also the DSM—which is a disaster, of course! Worst of all, perhaps, are the drug companies: they have so much power in America, it's unbelievable. In France as well.

TW: Could you point out more challenges in life, or in suffering? Or in questions of sexuality, as sexuality is at the core of psychoanalysis. If we think of transgender questions: do you think that there are any problems for psychoanalytic theory to answer those questions in any way? Or does the map fit the landscape, so to speak?

BF: Of that, I'm not sure, but I have a friend and colleague, Patricia Gherovici, who works on transgender issues from a Lacanian perspective. I think that Lacanian theory probably has more to say about gender trouble and transgender issues than a lot of conventional psychoanalysis does, which often doesn't want to go near such questions. I think that we're perhaps better equipped to address such questions than other approaches owing to Lacan's later work on the formulas of sexuation and the sinthome.[2]

I think more work should be done in Lacanian circles on so-called eating disorders, which are rampant in the United States. Eating problems of one kind or another are perhaps what lead the most young women, but some young men as well, to be sent to horrible inpatient treatment facilities. Lacanians rarely advertise that they specialize in any specific sort of problems—for example, phobias, impotence, marital conflict, anxiety, or what have you—and have no reputation for treating eating problems. But they probably have a lot to say about them and a good deal of success treating them. Yet there isn't much literature in the Lacanian world on those topics. There probably should be. We tend to look at eating problems as just one symptom among others, while the public tends to focus on symptoms when they go in search of a therapist, trying to find someone who specializes in their particular symptom. I've heard therapists say, "You can't send people with eating disorders to Lacanians because they don't know what to do." I don't think that's true, but it's something we rarely talk about publicly, much less write books about that might come to the attention of a broader reading public.

TW: It's interesting that you said you think there needs to be some work done on this specific topic. Has the lack of writings on the subject anything to do with the phenomenon as such?

BF: Therapists who treat eating problems are often looking for literature that might help them figure out how to handle them. There are a few articles in French that I've seen, but I know of no Lacanians who have written books about them.[3] Practitioners who know nothing about Lacan might happen upon a book that purports to talk about the treatment of anorexia and bulimia. That might somehow bring them into a more Lacanian way of thinking, or even just help them with their work with other people.

TW: Can you say something more about what patients come to you?

BF: Because of the peculiarities of my own practice, being a Lacanian in private practice and also probably because I've written and translated a lot, I tend to have a very highly educated population. They aren't always of high socio-economic status—indeed, rarely so—but they're people who have a master's degree at a minimum. Over the years, I have had a lot of doctors, clinicians, and professors on my couch. People who work in other professions come to me, too, but they've often studied Lacan in college at some point. This is not true of every Lacanian in the United States, of course. Patricia Gherovici had a job for a number of years working in a low-income and mostly Puerto Rican neighborhood in the Philadelphia area, so she worked with people from many different walks of life, especially from very impoverished walks of life. The type of problems that the people who come to see me come with are all across the board; there's no regularity to the type of problems they have.

TW: The question of some kind of loneliness, is it addressed?

BF: It's addressed, certainly. Loneliness was one of the biggest things that brought people into therapy at the psychology clinic at the university where I taught, where the majority of the patients were under thirty. I was shocked over the years to see the real disintegration of people's families and lives, and to see that people live in such isolated manners today: no real friends, very little contact with their family, or that's their only contact and they feel very alienated from it. That was a very common complaint at our clinic, which is surprising because the college experience in the United States is reputedly a time when you make a ton of friends.

These little devices here [points at a mobile phone] have changed peoples' lives. Twenty-five years ago, when I would teach a class, over the course of the semester the students would get to know each other's names, they would talk with each other, they would become friends, and they would go and have lunch together after class. By the time I left teaching, nobody talked to anybody anymore in class. The students would come in, look at their phones, text their friends, look at Facebook, and so on. They no longer knew how to talk with each other, they had become very awkward socially, and knew nothing of the social graces or politeness. If, in the course of a class discussion, they had to refer to something one of the other students had said, instead of using his name, they would say, "What *he* said," and I would have to remind them that *he* has a name. There's something new and different going on with human beings.

PL: Does that in any way change the preconditions for the psychoanalytic encounter?

BF: Yes, sure. What I think has started to happen in the States is that even the people who are now training as analysts are afraid of certain kinds of human contact. France is very refreshing to me because people always shake hands with each other and kiss each other—there's a lot more physical contact. The same is true in Italy. But in America, people are increasingly distant and cold, afraid of human contact and awkward about it. They don't know how to do things with other people anymore.

TW: So there is some kind of fear.

BF: Yes, and I think it also has to do with a kind of isolation growing up. There are more and more children growing up today in families where there's only one child, maybe two. Sometimes the families are very fragmented. They don't learn how to get along with other children very early on in life. When they're with other children, they're either very aggressive or they get precociously sexual. Some things that would have been taken for granted earlier in time, when there were more children in each family and there were more connections between different families, aren't there. Now, in America, people move on average every year and a half. That's a scary statistic. Jobs send people across the country, or to other countries, all the time now. If you make friends in a certain place and then move a year and a half later, you probably lose most of those friends. You keep up with them for a while, and Facebook gives you the illusion that you can keep up with them as long as you like. But is there much real contact? No, there's a lot less. In the end you don't have anybody but yourself anymore. American society is being atomized and it's very concerning. In the end, your therapist becomes your best friend because he's the only person you see regularly!

PL: Do you think psychoanalysis can, in a metaphorical sense, help break the screen and open up the dimension of the encounter?

BF: I'm not sure. Maybe it can help break down some of the fears that people have about social contact with other people. But it would be a lot easier if social contact was plentiful right from the outset.

TW: If we believe that psychoanalysis has something to say about what it is to be a social human being, and therefore also has something to say about contemporary loneliness—the lack of symbolic structures as one major part of the changes in society—would it be a reasonable thought that we who are interested in this should also work harder to be closer to some kind of majority society, in order to have a greater influence on the culture?

BF: You mean like being involved in political movements?

TW: Political movements, or maybe at the university which has been this struggle you talk about, where psychoanalysis really hasn't gotten its place. Is it sometimes too comfortable to maintain a certain distance to these realities? Or is it necessary for psychoanalysis to be a bit of an outsider?

BF: Both. I think it's good for psychoanalysis to be rejected in certain ways by mainstream discourse because it makes it more attractive to certain people who are disaffected, who don't feel accepted or welcomed by mainstream discourse and who are rebelling against it. I think that's potentially a good thing for psychoanalysis. The more psychoanalysis becomes part of mainstream discourse, the more it loses its critical edge and becomes invested in certain kinds of power structures that perhaps subtly but insidiously change the theory and practice itself.

On the question of what sort of movements analysts could support to try to counter the devastating things that are happening in our time (and wow, there are so many of them!): how could you get psychoanalysts to agree on a political platform when it's so hard to get two psychoanalysts to agree with each other about anything and work together in a psychoanalytic training institute? To try to give psychoanalysis a place in universities is a worthwhile endeavor. At the same time, not having the university stamp of approval can be a good thing. But it is important to have at least some representation there because that is how many people come to find out about psychoanalysis. Lacan talks about the incompatibility between psychoanalytic discourse and university discourse, and there's a lot of truth to that. Nevertheless many people become fascinated by psychoanalysis because they hear about it in college. I was happy when I left Duquesne because they actually hired Derek Hook, a prominent Lacanian, to take my place—that was unbelievable!

CHAPTER 11

A Lacanian approach to Freud

(Interview conducted by Tiago Gandra, M.D., in Copenhagen on April 15, 2018. Published in the Newsletter of the Faculty of Medical Psychiatry at the Royal College of Psychiatrists, London, Summer/Autumn 2018.)

Tiago Gandra (TG): I thought we could begin by talking about your most recent book, *A Clinical Introduction to Freud: Techniques for Everyday Practice*, in which you set out to revisit some classic Freudian ideas, bringing them to life in the consulting room. Was this a "return to Freud" for you, or has Freud's work always been central to your clinical practice?

Bruce Fink (BF): More the latter, I'd say. The book was based on semester-long undergraduate and graduate courses that I taught at Duquesne University for twenty years, so for me it was not a "return" to Freud. I have been reading Freud's texts for over forty years, and they have informed all of my work. While most of my writing was devoted to presenting Lacan to an English-reading audience, my teaching always included Freud. It was only when I decided to leave the university that I thought I might be able to do something interesting with all the course notes I had, which reflected much of the work I had done on Freud over the years. In many American training institutes Freud was being forgotten, or at least less often read seriously, and I felt it was important to reintroduce Freud to clinicians. That is why I tried to focus the book on very practical techniques that can be used every day; I did not want to delve into "heady" Freudian theory, but to take things in a rather more clinical direction.

TG: You mentioned the American context in particular, but do you think there is a risk of Freud being forgotten in training institutes worldwide? Or is it rather the case that clinicians and academics will continue arguing with Freud, even when they are doing so following a conceptual map that was largely drawn by Freud himself?

BF: I can't answer that question for the whole world, but it seemed to me that there was a risk, especially as of five or ten years ago, that Freud and psychoanalysis as a whole would be systematically eliminated from psychology training programs. Clinical psychology programs seemed to be completely uninterested in Freud, as did most psychiatry programs. Even in psychoanalytic institutes it was rare to come across someone who had actually read *The Interpretation of Dreams* from cover to cover. Now something of a sea change appears to be taking place, and I have been hearing more often about people who are starting to read Freud and to teach Freud at institutes.

Indeed, there was a point at which people were still implicitly arguing against Freud. But if people stop reading Freud for a long enough period of time, that generation will eventually die out, and the new generation will have little or no interest in his work. I think there is a growing interest in Lacan in the United States, which is driving a renewed interest in Freud, but there are probably other reasons of which I am unaware for the current return to Freud. In any case, it's a good sign!

TG: In this book you chose to give particular emphasis to Freud's early work on hysteria, dream interpretation, obsession, and the Freud of the first topography, so to speak. Is this because it is there that the focus on language and discourse, so central to the Lacanian tradition, stands out the most?

BF: I especially wanted to emphasize Freud's early work because that is the work that I myself find most clinically useful. His later works—such as *The Ego and the Id*, *Civilization and Its Discontents*, and *Moses and Monotheism*—all contain intriguing ideas and theory, but they don't seem to me to be immediately relevant to clinical practice.

TG: I suspect that in the UK, some analysts might argue that the structural model [i.e., the second topography] has been particularly helpful in working with patients presenting with a non-neurotic pathology. There is a sense of a different population of patients walking into consulting rooms these days presenting with a different clinical picture where the textual dimension and the metaphorical nature of symptoms seems to be less prominent.

BF: I am not so sure of that. I am always a bit skeptical of trend-spotters. In France there are people who have declared "the death of interpretation," that symptoms are no longer what they used to be, and so on, but I don't buy that personally. I think there are changes for sure, things are evolving, but the idea that there is a radical break in the way subjectivity is structured—I just don't see that in my own consulting room day in and day out.

TG: In brief, and bearing in mind that many clinicians reading this interview will have been trained in the British school of object relations, what would you say is most distinctive about a Lacanian approach to Freud?

BF: Many things, of course. But the one that comes to mind right now is that Lacan emphasizes something that is clearly there in Freud's work, but which seems to have been largely overlooked. People tend to emphasize the *meaning* of the things that Freud talked about, but not his attention to the *letter*. People are far more interested, for instance, in the Oedipus complex, drives, and the superego than in the way Freud actually worked, the way he paid attention to speech, language, double-entendres, slips of the tongue, and so on. Much of what Freud tells us about the way he himself practiced seems to have taken a back seat to his theoretical views. Personally, I find that the theories and models of the mind he constructed are of less enduring interest than the actual practice he helped develop. Lacan does not exactly endorse Freud's topographical models. He examines them, talks about them, and plays with them; but you rarely see Lacan truly take them up in his own name. Freud's clinical method, however, is something he uses a great deal.

TG: In the UK there has been a rich dialogue with the "French school" of psychoanalysis in recent years, and with that a renewed interest in some key Lacanian ideas. It is not unusual to hear references to, for instance, the "mirror stage" in the emergence of subjectivity; or a reference to the "Name-of-the-Father" when discussing an aspect of paternal functioning. Other central concepts of

Lacanian theory have not gained the same traction. Why do you think that is?

BF: It's hard for me to respond because in the United States, for instance, my sense is that people in the psychoanalytic community have often heard of the mirror stage but don't have any clear understanding of what it means, and often simply confuse it with Winnicott's notion of mirroring. As for the Name-of-the-Father, they may have heard the expression but generally don't know much about it, and when they do they usually don't endorse it because the Lacanian conception of a radical difference between neurosis and psychosis is foreign to them. They have a very fluid view of psychopathology, such that one and the same person can be sometimes neurotic and sometimes psychotic. "Borderline" is a major category for them, and it is incompatible with the theory built around the Name-of-the-Father. I don't have the impression that Lacan's work has been even the slightest bit assimilated by the psychoanalytic community in the U.S.

Let me point out that the two notions you mentioned—the mirror stage and the Name-of-the-Father—are theoretical, not clinical. They can inform clinical practice but have little to do with what one actually does in the consulting room. They have nothing to do with how one employs time, as in the use of *scansion* to create variable-length sessions, or the way one *punctuates* words or phrases, or how one might interpret from a Lacanian perspective. Just as with Freud's work, people are fascinated by Lacan's theory, but pay little attention to his approach to practice. Interestingly, Lacan was kicked out of the IPA not because of his theory but because of his practice!

TG: For the uninitiated, who know very little of Lacanian theory or practice, reading Lacan can be a really daunting exercise. What advice would you give them? Where should people begin?

BF: I always advise people to read the Seminars, beginning with Seminar I. They should certainly *not* begin with the *Écrits*. In the English-speaking world, *The Four Fundamental Concepts of Psychoanalysis* (Lacan, 1978a) was the first seminar to be translated, but it was presented as a stand-alone book, which it certainly is not, rather than as the eleventh seminar. Had it been presented as Seminar XI, people might have realized that there were ten years of seminars that preceded it, about which they knew nothing, and that might have helped explain why it was so difficult! How can anyone possibly understand the eleventh year of somebody's course without having attended the first ten years? In any case, the first seminars have now been quite competently translated into English, so why not begin there? They allow for an at least relatively easy introduction to his work.

What people should know when they later decide to tackle the *Écrits* is not to get bogged down on the first page or two of any one article. Lacan often made the first couple of pages of his texts impenetrably dense, but they get easier after that. Lacan had a penchant for making the reader's task as difficult as possible; we have to be careful not to fall into his trap by being scared off by a couple of cryptic pages.

TG: That reflects Lacan's suspiciousness of definite explanations and clear understanding. He was more comfortable with ambiguity and equivocation.

BF: For sure, but those are not the only reasons why the reader's task is a difficult one. I think Lacan both wanted to be understood and didn't want to be understood. He wanted to slap a lot of people in the face and say, "If you haven't read as much poetry and philosophy as I have, you can't possibly follow my work." Thus it is only those who are undaunted by the first pages and feel they can actually understand a little bit who tend to go on and continue to read. Like Plato, perhaps, Lacan was only willing to be understood by those whom he considered to be "worthy."

CHAPTER 12

Why Freud? Why psychoanalysis?

(Interview conducted by Mihaela Bernard via email. It appeared in the electronic magazine *Mental Health Digest* on April 11, 2017.)

Mihaela Bernard (MB): Dr. Fink, thank you for agreeing to do this interview. It is an honor to be able to talk to you about psychoanalysis and your new book.
Bruce Fink (BF): Thank you! It is an honor for me to be asked.
MB: For those who do not know you, can you tell us a little bit about yourself and what you do?
BF: I acquired a broad background in the sciences and the humanities—having studied math, physics, literature, psychology, political theory, and philosophy for many years—before doing my graduate work in Paris, where I simultaneously trained as a psychoanalyst. I taught psychoanalysis in the Department of Psychology at Duquesne University in Pittsburgh, Pennsylvania, for twenty years, and have been practicing psychoanalysis for

over thirty years, writing many books about it and translating several works by Jacques Lacan, the famous French psychoanalyst, into English. I have a very international practice, and divide my time between the U.S. and France. In more recent years, I have been cultivating anew my love for literature by dabbling in the writing of novels—mysteries involving an inspector loosely based on Lacan who solves crimes using psychoanalytic methods!

MB: How did you discover psychoanalysis and what attracted you to it?

BF: I became interested in psychoanalysis in my late teens as a way of trying to understand myself and the people around me. I became fascinated by the emphasis on the unconscious in the work of Jacques Lacan and decided to undergo analysis with a Lacanian in Paris in the 1980s.

MB: Tell us about your new book. What gave you the idea to write *A Clinical Introduction to Freud*?

BF: What, one might wonder, could there possibly be left to say about Freud that hasn't already been said by dozens of writers? Much to my surprise, and despite having taught Freud's work for over twenty years to undergraduate and graduate students at Duquesne University, I never came across any book that showed how to apply the techniques Freud developed to encourage free association and interpret dreams, for example. The vast majority of books on Freud seem to be devoted to expounding and/or criticizing his theories, or to talking about the personal, historical, and intellectual development of Freud the man.

My interest has always been in explaining those of Freud's ideas that are of direct use to practitioners and that seem to me to have survived the test of time. Whereas his speculations regarding the Oedipus complex, female sexual development, and the oral, anal, and genital stages tend to receive the lion's share of writers' attention in most textbooks and even in many advanced presentations of his work, these strike me as of little direct usefulness in the clinical setting. On the other hand, learning how to trace symptoms back to their sources, encourage patients to free associate to their stray thoughts, daydreams, and night dreams, and locate wishes in them can be of immense and immediate value to clinicians of many different persuasions.

I became convinced that this was so by seeing, over the course of two decades, how useful the class I gave on Freud was to graduate students in clinical psychology, helping them expand their array of techniques and deepen their psychotherapeutic practice more generally. Having once again surveyed the available literature recently and finding nothing that seemed to me specifically designed to present what is still clinically relevant in Freud's work today, I decided to turn my course into a book.

MB: Who would benefit from reading your new book?

BF: Any and all clinicians looking for ways in which to broaden and deepen their own practice. And especially those who are interested in the unconscious but whose training has never really taught them how to gain access to it.

MB: What would you say to the next generation of clinicians?

BF: Don't throw the baby out with the bathwater! Just because certain of Freud's more speculative theories have rightly been called into question and even sharply critiqued, that doesn't mean that the more fundamental concepts and techniques he developed related to the unconscious, free association, and dream interpretation are useless. Studies in France have shown that people who go through analysis often say that their work with dreams was the most helpful part of their analyses. I think we should take what patients say was most helpful to them very seriously indeed!

MB: Why psychoanalysis?

BF: I could approach this question from many different angles, but let me simply point out a very curious fact: when psychologists themselves decide to go into therapy—regardless of whether they are practitioners of CBT, cognitive psychology, existential phenomenology, hypnosis, or what have you—they almost invariably seek out a psychoanalyst. (This has been pointed out by many clinicians, although the evidence for it is largely anecdotal as no one seems to be willing to do a full-blown study of it.) There thus appears to be an implicit recognition of the value of in-depth psychoanalysis on the part of clinicians of virtually all ilks, even though many of them would dispute large swaths of psychoanalytic theory and even critique psychoanalytic practice in any and every public forum. When it comes to getting treatment for themselves, they seek out analysis. Go figure!

MB: In your opinion, who can benefit from a psychoanalytic treatment?

BF: It seems to me that this question cannot be answered in advance—that is, before someone begins treatment. A psychoanalysis is hard work and analysands must show courage and fortitude if they are to get something out of it.

Those who are looking for easy answers are not likely to go far in analytic treatment, but there are no hard and fast rules here: sometimes even people looking for quick fixes get intrigued by the process and end up going very far.

MB: How would you say psychoanalysis and the work you do as a psychoanalyst permeate your everyday life?

BF: Once you have learned to hear people's slips of the tongue and double entendres, you cannot turn such hearing off and inevitably notice slips and mistakes made by loved ones, friends, and even casual acquaintances. This can occasionally be awkward, but I try to turn such things into opportunities for good-natured levity.

Then there are, of course, the friends and family that come to you for advice, which is something an analyst should always avoid giving in the analytic setting, but which we sometimes feel obliged to give to family and friends, even if we know that this usually gives rise to a no-win situation for us: if the advice is taken and things work out, we are rarely credited for it, and if things don't work out, we are almost invariably blamed for it!

In a personal vein, psychoanalysis is an ongoing practice that keeps me aware of all kinds of things about myself, regardless of whether they arise while I am awake or asleep.

MB: Please share with our audience your writing process. What inspires you to write?

BF: I am always writing and each writing project is different. In the case of my book on Freud, I knew I had a lot of good material from my course, but I needed to find an angle that would inspire me to get started and organize the material. Once I found my angle—the exclusively clinical approach to Freud's work—everything else fell into place.

MB: What recommendations do you have for those of us who aspire to write about psychoanalysis?

BF: Don't wait until you think you have thought something out completely. The writing process itself puts your thinking to the test in a way that thinking things through in the privacy of your own head does not. This is related to what Lacan calls the Other with a capital O: simply stated it has to do with the fact that once you write up an idea, you can step back from it and try to look at it as other people might, at which point flaws in your argument or exceptions often spring to mind! It is probably an illusion to think you can work out all the details in your head before beginning to write. It is only by writing that you can begin to see what is going to be comprehensible and what is not going to be comprehensible to your intended audience. Steps and moves that seem obvious to you will not seem so to others, and the only way to realize that is to put it down on paper, set it aside for a while, and come back to it with fresh eyes.

Even better, of course, is to give a draft to trusted colleagues to read and take their points of view seriously! I gave this *Clinical Introduction to Freud* to a half-dozen friends and colleagues to read and they provided hundreds of incredibly useful comments that allowed me to vastly improve the book.

MB: Any final thoughts?

BF: Is there anything final about psychoanalysis? Can there be such a thing as a last word?!

MIS-CALCULATIONS

CHAPTER 13

Comments at the book launch for *A Clinical Introduction to Freud* (2017)

(Duquesne University, October 26, 2017.)

I'd like to thank Jim Swindal and Derek Hook for organizing this book launch and thank everyone for joining us here this evening. It is fitting for this particular book to be launched at Duquesne, since it is largely based on course materials I developed during my twenty years of teaching here.
    I have to admit that I hesitated for a while before deciding to write it, not being sure the world had any use for or interest in yet another book on Freud. I wasn't sure, either, if I could find the necessary starting point that would allow me to organize hundreds of pages of undergraduate and graduate class notes into a readable whole with a logic of its own.
    Shortly after I found my entry point—that is, the initial direction in which I wanted to take the book—the editor at W. W. Norton & Company with whom I had worked on an earlier book (*Fundamentals of Psychoanalytic Technique*), called me up out of the blue and asked if I was writing anything new. When I told her what it was,

she immediately asked me to send her what I had, and within a week I had a contract in hand, with the sole verbal recommendation to keep adding clinical examples of my own to what was already a rather clinically oriented book.

The reception the book has thus far had is surprising to me. Published in March 2017, the book was almost instantaneously put on the syllabi of Freud courses at a dozen psychoanalytic institutes, and within six months was under contract to be translated into Greek, Japanese, Chinese, Korean, Portuguese, Turkish, and German!

Although I have devoted several decades to translating Lacan's work and writing about it, none of my prior books have ever taken off like this one. It seems as though, unbeknownst to me, analytic training programs were just dying to find someone willing to brave the Freud-bashing of the past thirty plus years—that is, the obsession in our times with Freud as a flawed individual, a misogynist, and a privileged, upper-middle class doctor—and re-center discussion of Freud on his relevance to clinical practice today.

Much, if not all, of the Freud-bashing has focused on the following:

1. Freud's social and religious extraction. Note that this is something of which we are all guilty: we all come from somewhere, are born into a certain family, religion, economic stratum, etc.
2. His personal flaws as both an individual and a practitioner. But aren't we all terribly flawed, in ways that we perhaps try to keep others from knowing about, but which if subjected to tremendous scrutiny, might discredit us considerably in others' eyes? I, for one, would hardly relish the thought that everything I'd ever done or said would be gone over with a fine-tooth comb and rendered public the way Freud's words and actions have been over the past hundred years, including papers and letters that he requested his family burn! Can you imagine if every email you ever wrote, every text you ever sent, every phone call you ever made, and all of your internet searches were made public?

Like many others, I prefer it when a theorist's life and practice seem to corroborate or fit his or her theory, but I suspect that few well-known thinkers can boast that their personal lives match the ideals they espouse in their written work or that would seem to grow out of or square with their theories. To mention just a few with whom you may be familiar:

1. Martin Heidegger, who was a known Nazi sympathizer.
2. Jean-Jacques Rousseau, who dropped off a number of his illegitimate children at charitable institutions, where they might either be cared for or die.
3. Jacques Derrida, who, according to my sources, cheated on his wife with virtually all of his female translators and slept with so many of his graduate students in the U.S. and France that I don't believe anyone can have an accurate count.
4. Jacques Lacan, who in a sense stole Georges Bataille's wife, and then cheated on her with myriad mistresses, and seems to have been a less-than-ideal father to at least one of his daughters.
5. Soren Kierkegaard (notice I've only mentioned Europeans), whose fascinating notions about Christian love might be called into question by an incredibly neurotic relationship to the love of his life, Regina.

The list goes on and on. If we knew a great deal more about Plato, Aristotle, Julia Kristeva, Judith Butler, and just about any other prominent figure, we might feel the need to either (1) accept the fact that seriously flawed individuals nevertheless sometimes have useful ideas, or (2) consign virtually everyone's work to the dustbin of history. Each of us has to make his or her own choice about that.

I, for one, have never been interested in Freud's life, or in Lacan's life for that matter. I've always been far more interested in theorists' ideas than in their lifestyles and personal trajectories.

And whether or not Freud himself was a good clinician has always struck me as something of a moot point. Freud himself admitted in myriad places in his work that he was unable to stop himself from doing many of the things he recommended that we *not* do—for example, give interpretations when people aren't ready to hear them (they should be only one short step away from formulating them themselves, he wrote). In many cases, he didn't give people time to really go into their own history and formulate things for themselves, as he was too impatient; for he admits to having wanted to spread his influence by working with as many future practitioners as possible—which is a travesty, really—and continued to act as though patients should change just by his depositing in them, as it were, knowledge that he felt *he* had arrived at of them, as if he could simply transfer his supposed knowledge to them and watch the happy results unfold. This was something he had repeatedly found to be ineffective and even cautioned against in his written work! He recommended, moreover, that we be mirrors, merely reflecting back to patients what they say, yet he kept bringing himself in—telling patients he, too, had phobias, for example!

Does the fact that Freud was not the best follower of his own theory of practice mean he wasn't on to something? Haven't there been practitioners since who have done a better job than Freud at marrying theory and practice, who have helped generations of patients? Is all of psychoanalytic practice to be impugned just because Freud was smitten with Dora and couldn't stop himself from trying to show off and provide her dazzlingly complex, but useless, interpretations of everything she said, did, and dreamed? Or because he became spiteful and embittered when she left treatment?

Imagine a professor of dental surgery who invents a better method for doing root canals, but who is a klutz with a drill and butterfingers with small metal tools and modern adhesives. The students who train with her will probably do a better job with patients than she ever did!

Imagine a cook who concocts a delicious new dessert and publishes the recipe in a cookbook, but every time he makes it at his own restaurant, he can't stop himself from tinkering with it a little, adding a bit of this or that, having an irrepressible urge for creation, which ends up making it worse, not better. The sous-chefs he trains might get a Michelin star whereas he won't!

Those who are most inventive in our own field (as in certain others) often learn a great deal by trial, error, and accident—which is how most investigative endeavors proceed, regardless of what philosophers of science tell us. One of my favorite wine makers in France, Frédéric Broché, accidentally created one of his signature wines, *Blanc d'Hiver*, while having an especially enjoyable night with his wife (personal communication), and forgetting to go check on a vat of wine he intended to let cool down only a little, not to the point of putting a stop to the fermentation.

Those who experiment sometimes bequeath useful techniques to future generations, after having not always helped, and sometimes even harmed, their own patients, diners, or what have you.

Much as we'd like theory and practice to go hand-in-hand, they very often don't. A self-correcting, self-consistent praxis is an ideal few live up to, whether in the operating room, the classroom, the kitchen, or the consulting room. If people actually practiced what they preached and the result was horrendous, we could easily discredit their theories. Freud certainly didn't and my argument in this book is that we can do patients a great deal of good by following certain of Freud's recommendations about how to work with parapraxes of all kinds, whether slips of the tongue, pen, or keyboard, and bungled actions, and about how to work with dreams and fantasies, anxiety, phobias, and neuroses of all kinds.

I point out that Freud was not terribly conversant with psychosis, often failed to recognize it in his patients—which is still true of a great many clinicians today, I would suggest—and never found a useful clinical stance that was helpful to psychotics. That's fine. We all have to start somewhere, and no one understands everything or everyone. Other theorists and practitioners, like R. D. Laing and Lacan's students, have arguably done far better with psychotics than Freud ever did. Isn't that just the way it is? Psychoanalysis is not a one-size-fits-all endeavor—rather it is a one-size-fits-one approach. Every case is unique, and every practitioner has to tailor what he or she does in the attempt to help each new patient who comes along.

In the book itself, I argue that psychoanalysis can have the kind of enduringly positive effect on people that psychotropic medications can never hope to have. And I cover some of the most basic Freudian notions and techniques:

1. That to have an impact on a symptom—which is something a person complains of, not something an outsider (whether a family member or psychologist) thinks is wrong with that person—we have to trace it back to its origins, to the best of our ability, and probably not just on one occasion, in one session, but in many. We have to explore all of the forces that were at work at the outset, many of which are probably still at work and hold the symptom in place.
2. That what we unconsciously think and desire is very often the exact opposite of what we consciously think and desire.
3. That what we fear and hate tells us a great deal about what we secretly desire and love.
4. That dreams fulfill wishes that we would rather not know about.

5. That what we think most disgusts us is often what we are most intrigued and even turned on by.
6. That we often end up repeating in our own lives—albeit unwittingly—the very things we are so critical of in our parents' lives.
7. That many people derive a great deal of satisfaction from complaining and that what they complain about most bitterly is often what they secretly most enjoy or can't live without.
8. That genuinely transformative self-analysis is structurally impossible; we need another person to be present, so as not to content ourselves too quickly with the first explanation we come up with, and so that this other person can hold the place of our unconscious for us.

CHAPTER 14

Introduction to Seminar VI

(These brief remarks were made, at the invitation of Derek Hook, at the *Écrits* conference held at Duquesne University on October 11–13, 2019.)

When, after publishing Seminar VIII, I proposed to Polity Press to translate Seminar XVI or XVIII, they countered that they had already contracted with the French publisher to bring out Seminar VI. The fact that Seminar VI was a bit boring to me, being old hat, cut no ice with the editors at Polity—they had, after all, just managed to negotiate a publishing agreement with the French, which is no mean feat! In the end, I agreed to translate Seminar VI if Polity promised to let me do Seminars XVI and XVIII when they became available. They promised and I set to work on *Desire and Its Interpretation*.[1]

Rereading the Seminar now with a year's distance, it seems to me to contain a number of useful reminders regarding desire, and regarding the interpretation of desire in dreams specifically.

Desire is defined here as something that arises for us assuming that we have gone beyond "being in the grip of language" (p. 14), assuming that we have come to inhabit language in a full-fledged way in which our speech can never exactly capture what we mean to say, always saying more or less than we wish it would. Desire is, Lacan tells us here, "riveted to a certain linguistic function—that is, to a certain relationship between the subject and the signifying system" (p. 5). Desire arises for those of us who perceive the Other with a capital O as having a desire that is "obscure and opaque" (p. 17), yet intriguing and important, not something to be taken at face value. What does this Other want of me, we wonder? We don't take for granted what the Other *says* he wants of us, but wonder what he *really* thinks of us and wants from us, which may be light-years from what he says he thinks and wants.

Psychotics, on the other hand, take what their parents say they want at face value. It may be persecutory or not, but it does not constitute a question to them, it is not a source of endless speculation and wondering for them.

Desire is thus immediately situated here by Lacan as something characteristic of neurosis, not psychosis. The neurotic subject is "caught up in speech" and thus in a relationship to the Other as the locus of speech in which a signifier—the phallus—is always missing (p. 23). Whereas need and demand unfold in the lower part of the graph of desire, desire proper unfolds in the upper part.

The psychotic does not proffer statements like, "I am *not* saying that my boss pisses me off," nor does he say "I am *not* saying that you drive me crazy." Such formulations are incredibly common in neurosis, the neurotic denying the very thing that has come to mind, it having been able to come to mind precisely because it presents itself under erasure—that is, with a giant X over it, crossing it out. Lacan calls such negating "the most radical property of the signifier" (p. 80). Even as the neurotic "cancels out the signifier," he "perpetuates it indefinitely" (p. 80), Lacan claims.

What does it mean in Seminar VI to interpret the desire in a dream? It means to *situate the subject with respect to ignorance, castration, and death*! In the dream that Freud recounts about a man who dreams he sees his father and is distressed that his father is dead but doesn't know it, Lacan argues that the dreamer's desire is to *remain ignorant*, ignorant of the fact that, now that his father is dead, he himself is next in line to die (p. 96). The will not to know is perhaps best known to us from Lacan's Seminar XX, *Encore*, but we see its crucial role here already: the subject prefers to project his own ignorance onto the other, onto the dreamer's father in this case (onto Lenin in the case of Trotsky's dream, p. 115). Better that the other be ignorant and castrated than me!

This, Lacan tells us, keeps the dreamer at some distance from his own death wish (pp. 96–97).

Lacan also tells us here that affect is something that concerns "a certain stance the subject adopts with respect to being." We tend to think Lacan didn't broach this topic until the 1970s in *Television*, but here it is on page 141, in January 1959!

Since we are at Duquesne University this weekend, I thought I might mention that we find in this Seminar a phrase many professors in the psychology department here might find anathema: "the phenomenology of castration" (p. 100). I missed the opportunity, when I was teaching here, to give a course on the topic, and can only hope that someday Derek Hook will do so!

As for my method of working on the translation of the Seminar, it was the same as for Seminar VIII: I checked and rechecked the English against the French several times, which for me meant comparing the published French version to the stenography and several so-called pirate versions of the Seminar. This is, in my view, indispensable if one hopes to determine *what* to translate, as a number of things are patently missing or false in virtually all extant versions of the Seminar.

I was imprudent enough to indicate that I had examined all the other extant versions in the translator's note I wrote to accompany the translation. I was also so stupid as to indicate that I had silently corrected hundreds of mistakes found in the La Martinière edition, for this led the French to suppress virtually all of my translator's note and all forty pages of the endnotes I had prepared. These can now be found in the form of a free downloadable PDF file on Polity's website, if you click on "Show More" under the book description or scroll to the bottom of the Table of Contents. They can also be found on my own website, if you scroll down to the bottom of my library page.

In the PDF file, you will find that I thank a number of people for help with the translation, including my wife for help with the French, Rolf Flor, who is here with us today, for help with the German, and Matthew Baldwin for help with the Greek. I was sorry not to be allowed to include my heartfelt thanks to them in the book itself.[2]

CHAPTER 15

Brief remarks made at the 25th anniversary of *A Clinical Introduction to Lacanian Psychoanalysis*

(Celebrated at the conference "Lacan: Clinic & Culture" organized by Derek Hook at Duquesne University, October 14–16, 2022.)

I'd like to thank all of my former students who have spoken today for their heartwarming comments![1] They are among the graduate students who made my years at Duquesne worthwhile.

My *Clinical Introduction to Lacanian Psychoanalysis* was, naturally, criticized in some French circles for oversimplifying—which is undoubtedly true. But the criticism in some cases simply meant that it rendered accessible certain of Lacan's ideas to non-specialists (against all odds, it has been translated into a dozen languages), many Lacanians being careful to never be too clear, to always leave some conceptual wiggle room, to always leave the listener or reader perplexed. That can be useful in a context in which the more listeners and readers are perplexed, the harder they work.

I would argue that that context—assuming it was ever really widespread—is gone, that that moment in time has passed. (I am sure I was also vilified for occasionally using inexcusable terms like "therapy" and "psychotherapist," instead of "analysis" and "analyst.")

I'd like to make a plea here for clear expression and the avoidance of jargon. Even a term as simple as that of "clinic" has turned into a mystifying bit of Lacan-speak today (my apologies to Derek). What exactly is "the clinic of foreclosure," "the clinic of psychosis," or "the clinic of jouissance"? It certainly isn't the Menninger Clinic or the Tavistock. To most ordinary English speakers, "clinic" refers to a physical space or building. If we mean the "clinical structure of psychosis," then we should say that even if it's already hard to grasp for practitioners who don't believe in structures, but only in lists of fluctuating symptoms patients have for at least five days or two weeks. If we mean "clinical work with jouissance," we should say that, even if jouissance is already a baffling term to many. "The Borromean clinic" sounds, for example, like a hospital named for the Italian mathematician, not a clinical and diagnostic approach that takes into account how the three registers, real, symbolic, and imaginary, are tied together or fail to be tied together. (I won't even mention a usage of the French term *"clinique"* that I came across recently by Mickaël Peoc'h: *"une clinique de l'analyste partenaire du symptôme"*; just imagine what that would sound like in unimaginative English: "a clinic of the analyst partner of the symptom").

"The real of the body" is also quite a mystifying formulation one hears bandied about, whereas "the body as real," or "the body as material" (or as materiality) is a bit less so.

So my plea here is that we *try* not to be hermetic. I am thrilled that my former students at Duquesne who are here today have striven to follow this non-hermetic path!

Before ending this evening, I'd like to briefly mention a series of recent books that have taken the treatment of psychosis much further than I did in my *Clinical Introduction to Lacanian Psychoanalysis*: Jean-Claude Maleval's *Foreclosure of the Name-of-the-Father*, *The Logic of Delusion*, and *Landmarks of Ordinary Psychosis*; and Mickaël Peoc'h's *Elegant Solutions to Psychosis*. They are only available thus far in French (and perhaps Spanish), I'm afraid.[2]

MIS-LAID

CHAPTER 16

Review of Elisabeth Roudinesco's biography entitled *Jacques Lacan* (New York: Columbia University Press, 1997)

(Initially commissioned from me in 1997 by an art journal, this book review was deemed too inflammatory—or politically incorrect—to publish. A typical example, in my view, of the unwillingness on the part of American publishers to foster genuine intellectual debate.)

Elisabeth Roudinesco's purpose in writing this book is rather obscure. While she seems to want to celebrate Lacan's genius, she simultaneously traces all of his revolutionary concepts back to his own psychological conflicts. Readers must prepare themselves for the most reductionistic form of psychobiography: Lacan's theory of psychosis is "shown" to grow out of his own psychotic tendencies (Roudinesco does everything but explicitly diagnose Lacan as psychotic), his conception of the fundamentally paranoid structure of the ego out of his own paranoia, and so on.

This reduction is brought about by interpreting Lacan's theories in the most banal manner possible. For an "intellectual historian" who has by now devoted over 2000 pages to the history of psychoanalysis, Roudinesco doesn't seem to grasp the most elementary concepts of Freud's work, much less Lacan's. To provide but one example,

Lacan's thirty years of study of psychosis, leading to the development of the notion of the *Nom-du-Père* (usually translated as "Name-of-the-Father"), is reduced in Roudinesco's work to nothing more than the father's literal last name! It has nothing, to her mind, to do with the paternal prohibition (the father's "No!" enunciated in the context of the Oedipal conflict, leading to the separation of the child from its mother), the father's naming of the mother's desire or prohibiting of the child's desire for the mother, the father as name (that is, as a part of speech in the mother's discourse), or the name as father—all of which are clearly intended by Lacan and explicitly articulated in his writings and seminars. Roudinesco, in taking up Lacan's extensive work on Schreber's (1988) *Memoirs of My Nervous Illness*—discussed at length by Freud (SE XII) in his "Psychoanalytic Notes on an Autobiographical Account of a Case of Paranoia"—offers nothing but the notion that what is foreclosed (radically rejected) in Schreber's case is his father's last name: "Schreber." Nothing could be further from Lacan's argument!

This conceptual reduction then "allows" Roudinesco to link Schreber to Lacan because Lacan, it seems, at an early age hated his grandfather whose last name he bore. While the biographical facts that Lacan may have hated his paternal grandfather and thought his own father weak (the latter apparently allowed himself to be dominated by Lacan's grandfather) likely say something about Lacan's own neurotic symptoms prior to undergoing analysis in his thirties, they hardly prove him psychotic.

Reducing all of his most important insights to his life story, Roudinesco argues that the theory of the Name-of-the-Father resulted directly from the fact that Lacan was unable to give his last name to one of his daughters until she was about twenty years old. Roudinesco never for a moment considers the fact that, unlike myriad other men who have been unable to pass on their last name to a child born out of wedlock, Lacan was the only one who developed a comprehensive theory of psychosis based on the father qua name and as the one who prohibits a potentially over-close relationship between mother and child (male or female).

While supposedly a sophisticated, fair-minded account of a great psychoanalytic thinker, Roudinesco's biography is marked by her considerable ambivalence regarding Lacan: on the one hand, she is completely captivated by the charisma and intellectual dazzle of this greatest of twentieth-century thinkers (as she calls him); but, on the other, she clearly ridicules him as a space-cadet—referring to him, for example, as an inhabitant "of the planet Borromeo," a planet where people presumably discourse upon such topological figures as the Borromean knot, which Lacan uses to illustrate the interconnectedness of his three registers (the imaginary, symbolic, and real), but which Roudinesco seems unable or unwilling to fathom. None of her obvious fascination with Lacan's thought that came through in her *Jacques Lacan & Co.* (1990, an abridged version of her voluminous *L'histoire de la psychanalyse en France*, 1986) is present here, and Lacan is simply asserted to be a brilliant mind, without Roudinesco indicating how or why he was so brilliant. Instead she ruthlessly defames him, adducing every possible contradiction between his theoretical work and his personal life, her whole intent in this book seeming to be to cast aspersions on Lacan's integrity as an analyst.

This contrasts sharply with the first-hand accounts—transcribed in her book verbatim on pages 392 to 397—given by people who were in analysis or supervision with Lacan toward the end of his life which attest to his sensitivity and receptiveness, as well as to his well-founded approach to practice. As Houda Aumont, one of his patients, says, "he had a fantastic ear for listening to people, a human approach that was very tactful and sensitive: I always felt he understood my suffering and wasn't looking down on me" (p. 393). Claude Halmos, one of his supervisees, offers the following: "He generally avoided giving hard and fast explanations and laying down the law about the 'best way' to do things. He tried to find out what made me tick and made me become an analyst through discovering my own 'style,' so to speak" (p. 395). Although these first-hand accounts also indicate that Lacan had become rather hard of hearing and irritable by 1978, they reveal just how helpful he was to his analysands and supervisees prior to that time, and hardly vitiate the preceding fifty years of clinical work.

In Part IX of the book it finally becomes clearer why Roudinesco wrote this account: while fascinated with Lacan's life and thought, she nevertheless can't countenance a particular interpretation thereof put forward by Lacan's son-in-law, Jacques-Alain Miller, who Lacan entrusted with the task of editing his work and heading a Lacanian school. Miller is taxed by her with having "made an oversimplified and reductive interpretation of Lacan's work" (p. 439), of having confused "legal rights and scientific debate" (p. 423), and of tolerating "no doctrinal divergences" (p. 433). Whether one agrees with her or not about these matters, one may well wonder what this discussion is doing in a biography of Jacques Lacan!

Indeed, the last section of Roudinesco's book is no more than a diatribe against Miller, a man largely unknown to the American reading public who has offered one of the few truly intelligible accounts of Lacan's work to date. Roudinesco seems to disapprove of the very clarity with which Miller has elaborated the logic of Lacan's teaching in his ongoing weekly seminar entitled "Orientation lacanienne." Hence she unwittingly idolizes the master's work in the purest form, preferring Lacan's deliberate obscurantism to any comprehensibly elaborated psychoanalytic theory.

Although Roudinesco laments the absence of good scholarship and adequate critical apparatus in Miller's published editions of Lacan's seminars, she herself provides an extremely flawed bibliography and footnotes. In the French edition, her page references, dates, and volume numbers are incorrect at least half the time; the percentage is quite a bit better in the English edition thanks to the heroic efforts of the editorial staff of Columbia University Press, who were smart enough to seek outside assistance.[1] Perhaps worst of all is Roudinesco's tendency to criticize out of hand what she so patently does not understand—hardly good scholarship—including all of Lacan's later work on logic, topology, and knots. Try as she might, Roudinesco is sure to never become an inhabitant of the "planet Borromeo" where citizens must have at least some knowledge of knot theory.

MIS-GUIDED

CHAPTER 17

A few notes on supervision

(This short piece is based on discussions held at the Pittsburgh Psychoanalytic Center, jointly with, and at the invitation of, Howard Foster, M.D., on December 5 and 12, 2018.)

When one has been asked to supervise someone, a good place to start is, I think, to inquire what he or she wants from supervision. Further preliminary questions include what he or she thinks worked and what did not in past supervisory experiences (if any); what he or she is struggling with and wants help with; and what he or she hopes to achieve, improve on, and learn. The question we as supervisors must then ask ourselves is: Can we provide what the supervisee is seeking or are we on different pages altogether?

I have found that, in many cases, people come asking for supervision, but soon conclude they need to go back into analysis. They had been hoping that a new approach to supervision would make up for something they feel they did not accomplish in their personal analyses. This can occasionally be glimpsed early on and is something the supervisor may be in a good position to draw them out about.

I, for one, don't view supervision as a continuation of one's own training analysis.[1] Serious personal problems that the supervisee has should be dealt with in his or her own analysis, not in supervision. To my way of thinking, supervision is above all designed to help analysts come to grips with their patients. That doesn't mean supervisees can't discuss with their supervisors their own parapraxes or dreams they have that are directly related to their patients. (Or that they can't discuss difficulties they are having with their analysis or training analyst; supervision seems, indeed, to be one of the only places people can discuss those.)

Insofar as supervision focuses primarily on the patients being seen by the supervisee, slips the latter makes during supervision can be viewed:

- As parapraxes to be taken up in his or her own analysis, or
- As a recognition or reflection of something about the patient under discussion—something the supervisee has noticed without noticing it consciously, or something the supervisee thought about bringing up but set aside.

I approach countertransferential reactions of the supervisee to the patient less in terms of the supervisee's own neurosis, than in terms of the way in which the supervisee is situating him- or herself in the treatment and the effects that is having on the patient.[2]

Some of the goals of supervision include collaborative work on:

- In the early stages: specific strategies for drawing the patient out, learning how to ask nonleading questions (like "What about that?" or "What do you make of that?" or "Can you say more about that?"), how to approach sensitive subjects, how to get the patient to associate to dreams, and how to begin to interpret them.
- In the more advanced stages: overall case formulation, including reconstruction of the patient's history, formulation of his or her fundamental fantasy, and of the patient's positioning in his or her life (that is, his or her "subjective position").

Supervisees' confidence in their supervisors depends on numerous factors, including whether the supervisor was assigned by their training program or freely chosen (based on transference to that person's knowledge or friendliness/cooperative spirit). Trainees often don't choose their first supervisor, but can choose later in their training and after their official training is complete. Later supervisory work differs in certain ways because the supervisee's competence and knowledge of most of the ethical conditions under which we work can be taken more or less for granted.

Things I try to stress

1) Supervision should generally be viewed as a lifetime endeavor, not something one does during one's four or more years of training and then abandons. We all need a forum in which to articulate our ongoing struggles with patients—especially those who seem not to be making progress or who are difficult for any other reason—and ongoing discussion of diagnosis, the best strategies for making the work move forward with specific patients, and so on.
2) Getting supervisees to think for themselves.
3) Helping supervisees develop their own styles.
4) Notetaking can be very distracting. Reliance on process notes in supervision can be useful for the nitty gritty blow-by-blow stuff, but writing down those notes takes therapists' minds off what they are doing. And it leads their patients to wonder what is going on, why the therapist is writing down everything, no matter how banal, or only what the therapist apparently thinks is important. Therapists should try to learn to recall almost verbatim certain exchanges: practice makes perfect (or almost). Freud wrote his notes on all of his cases at the end of the day; I'd recommend at the end of each session, so time needs to be left before the next patient arrives.

    Exclusive reliance on process notes in supervision can lead both parties to lose sight of the bigger picture: each interpretation should be made in light of the patient's entire history and the unfolding of the therapy.
5) It is important to bring not just one case to supervision, but many (assuming supervisees have many), even at the outset. This gives the supervisor a better idea of where supervisees are at, how they react to different patients, where they need work, theoretical and otherwise. Systematic blindness becomes visible, as it were, whereas it may remain invisible when only one case is discussed. It is important to encourage practitioners to bring the most difficult cases to supervision, the cases in which they feel they are doing a bad job or have screwed up, to counter the tendency on their parts to try to convince their supervisors that they are doing a good job—whether to graduate from their training programs, garner praise, or get future referrals.

An amusing anecdote

Phyllis Grosskurth (1987) reports that when Klein was supervising a young analyst by the name of Sonny Davidson who told her, "I interpreted to the patient that he put his confusion into me," Klein replied, "No dear, that's not it, *you* were confused!" (p. 449).

Grosskurth goes on to say that Klein "was particularly worried about the 'fashion' for countertransference she saw developing. If a candidate tended to talk too much about how a patient made him angry or confused, she would remark pithily: 'Look, you tell that to your analyst. I really want to know something about your patient'" (p. 449).

Self-disclosure

There is something symptomatic about the fact that one of the only extant papers on supervision in the non-Lacanian psychoanalytic literature (Weinstein, Winer, & Ornstein, 2009) focuses on self-disclosure—self-disclosure by both the supervisee and the supervisor.[3] There seems to me to be a gnawing sense in psychoanalytic circles that there is something not quite kosher about self-disclosure.

What can we say about the current obsession with self-disclosure? I would propose that it is a symptom of the fact that analysts want to be loved by their analysands for themselves, rather than for the fact that they play a disciplined role with patients that provides certain intellectual gratifications, but few, if any, opportunities to talk about themselves and express their feelings. Psychoanalysis gives us analysts a chance to develop our individual discursive styles—which may involve playfulness, poetry, dialectic, and so on—but not a chance to blow off steam, get things off our chests, or "be ourselves" (whatever that means).

What self-disclosive analysts seem to be doing is taking a situation that is fundamentally not about them and making it about them. Some analysts try to relate everything patients say to themselves, even when it is a real stretch. Every dream has to be made about the analyst, even when the connection is quite far-fetched. People who engage in self-disclosure should realize that all speech, especially about oneself, is a request to be loved, in this case, loved for oneself, one's feelings, one's reactions, and one's so-called intuitions. We should *not* be asking the patient to love us![4]

Self-disclosure makes it harder for patients to say what they have to say, because they know more about you, or think they do, and end up tailoring what they say to who they think you are, what you are willing and not willing to hear, and so on. It is an illusion to believe that self-disclosure introduces "reality" into the analysis, or that it forces analysands to deal with the "real you," because you, too, are a divided subject and do not fully know yourself.

One-off supervision

When I lecture at analytic institutes, I am often asked to comment publicly on a case presented by a trainee at the institute (full members are rarely willing to present in front of such groups, in my experience, for a variety of complex reasons, I suspect). As opposed to requesting process notes from one or two sessions from the trainee, which is what often seems to be done, this is the request I usually send regarding his or her upcoming presentation (which I request he or she send me at least a couple of days in advance so I can familiarize myself with the case):

> What I would hope for from you would be a case write-up, complete with some detailed family history, early childhood experiences, important turning points in the patient's history, "presenting problems" and other symptoms that have surfaced over the course of the therapy, developments over the course of the therapy, whether transferential or changes of whatever sort, blockages/stagnation, perhaps a dream or two, and fantasies. I would hope you would speak for about forty-five minutes or so and then we would devote at least an hour to discussing the case, trying to figure out together what is going on or failing to go on, hypothesizing about diagnosis, the patient's fundamental fantasy, keys to his or her symptoms, the positioning of the analyst in the case, and so on.

MI(S)-DIRE

CHAPTER 18

Afterthoughts: maxims and quotes

In psychoanalysis, we know what happens, not why.

You know you've really entered into analysis when you realize you're full of shit.

Trying to get back what you think you've lost leads you to lose everything—even what you haven't yet lost.

Timing is incredibly important in comedy and psychoanalysis.

The couch is a wild and wonderful place. One can *lose* one's wallet in it, one's bus or subway pass, one's loose change, one's comb, one's guitar pick, or any number of other objects like hairbands, keys, or papers with phone numbers on them. But one can also *find* things there: relief, tears, laughter, freedom.

We wish to be what we most profoundly sense we are not.

Nothing hurts quite like the truth.

The best interpretation you ever made is one you don't remember. (And even if you could, your analysand probably remembers it differently.)

In psychoanalysis, there's no such thing as a *non sequitur*.

The notion of "boundary violations" is for those who wouldn't know a boundary if it bit them in the ass.

There's no fun in fundamentalism.

In France one can only enjoy through transgression of the law.

Anyone who hasn't been analyzed is only half alive.

Love is giving what you never really received.

Ye who seek praise from analysands for serving as their analyst are in the wrong profession.

Women want someone *qui les fait vibrer*, men want someone *qui les fait bander*.

Object relations theory attracts people with poor object relations.

In France, you never really deserve anything you have: you are guilty of having money, property, and the rest. You can only enjoy it surreptitiously as a guilty pleasure. In the U.S., you are allowed to enjoy what you have earned.

Men want to piss off other men.

It's not enough to say that others are prisoners of some narrow way of thinking to avoid falling into that same way of thinking oneself.

To break the rules, you must first master them.

Une femme, ça ne s'invente pas.

Le boire est le propre de l'homme.

I, of course, haven't had the time to say everything, so, as long as I'm alive, don't think you can take any of my formulations to be definitive—I still have other little things up my sleeve [or: in my bag of tricks, *sac à malices*].
 —Jacques Lacan ("Petit discours aux psychiatres," a lecture given on November 10, 1967, unpublished)

As a therapist, it's not about what you bring, it's about what you leave behind.
 —An analysand

I haven't discovered anything. I've only found out what I know.
 —Tolstoy

In a time of universal deceit, telling the truth becomes a revolutionary act.
 —Orwell

Les malades sont moins bêtes que les psychanalystes. (Patients are less dumb than psychoanalysts.)
 —Jacques Lacan (Seminar XIV, p. 304)

ENDNOTES

Chapter 1: On the value of the Lacanian approach to analytic practice

1. Analysts trained by Freud and Lacan have perhaps at times proven to be better practitioners than either Freud or Lacan was.
2. He adds puns to slips of the tongue in the next breath.
3. One might add "schizoaffective" to the list.
4. Concerning Lacanian approaches to work with psychotics, see ECF, 1997a, 1997b, 2005; and Fink, 2007, chapter 10. See, also, Chapter 2 in the present volume.
5. I usually try to vary male and female pronouns in my writing, or formulate things in the plural so as to avoid singular pronouns altogether, but this was discouraged by the *IJP*.
6. So-called body language is not viewed as transparently understandable, it being so culturally specific and individual; it cannot be "read" directly by the analyst, but must be spoken about (which is not to say that all speech is naïvely assumed to be truthful and straightforward—far from it!). Nor do I know of any Lacanians who believe we pick up on what analysands are feeling via pheromones, something I have heard

from a number of American analysts (see my comments on this in Fink, 2016, pp. 125–126).

7. Lacanian critiques of the use made of countertransference and of "projective identification" in other schools can be found in Miller, 2003, and Fink, 2007, chapter 7.
8. See Lacan, 1990; Soler, 2015, chapter 4. Note that the generally deluded belief that all will work out in the realms of love and sex *if one can simply meet the right person* is echoed in the oft-heard stress on "fit" in the analytic setting, it being thought by some that there must be "a good fit" between the (type of) patient and the (type of) analyst if the work is to proceed well.
9. See Lacan, *Écrits* and Seminar VIII; Fink, 2016.
10. If Chelsea understood at that early age what life insurance actually does and that Chelsea herself would have been the likely beneficiary of the policy, then we perhaps cannot even consider it to have been an unconscious death wish on her part.
11. There is nothing mysterious about how this happens (we have no need to resort to ideas like "projective identification" to explain it): if you tell someone over and over that he must be worried about something, you will sooner or later convince him that he is (or at least should be) worried about it.
12. Or we assist him in arriving at a different attitude or stance with respect to his symptoms, one in which he is less dissatisfied with the satisfactions he already has.
13. This sort of thing rarely, if ever, happens with psychotics, which is in part why Lacanians have, for the most part, stopped using the couch altogether with psychotics.
14. See Fink, 2007, chapters 3 and 5.
15. This paper was presented orally in a number of venues, including the daylong workshop entitled "Lacan's Revolution in Technique," sponsored by IPTAR in New York City on December 2, 2017; the daylong workshop on November 3, 2018 at the Dallas Society for Psychoanalytic Psychology; an open lecture at the University of Copenhagen on September 20, 2019; and the Hyman Fingert Lecture at the Saint Louis Psychoanalytic Society on October 4, 2019.
16. For a short list of books that indicate how different human gestures—whether hand, facial, or bodily—are in different cultures, see Chapter 3, "The Many Faces of the Imaginary."

17. I would nevertheless point out that, to the best of my knowledge, there has never been a law of the land, or a set of moral or religious laws, that does not stem—when we look at its origins—from something that precedes all law: a "just because (I/we said so)," whether that be the "just because" of the "founding fathers," of the God of the *Old Testament*, or of a parent in that parent's own home. All systems, including those based on a supposed "social contract" or lists of "human rights," can be questioned as to why we—who were not present at the hammering out of the contract and never agreed to the initial bill of rights—should adopt and obey them.
18. One might hypothesize that the importance of the "frame" is the only thing that the vast majority of non-Lacanian analysts still agree upon. Yet let us recall Winnicott's (1958b) comment about working with neurotics, in which I believe the term "setting" was used in much the same way as many use the term "frame" today: "Where there is an intact ego and the analyst can take for granted these earliest details of infant care, then the setting of the analysis is unimportant relative to the interpretive work. (By setting, I mean the summation of all the details of management)" (p. 297).

Chapter 2: Transference revisited: how neurotic and psychotic patients use us differently

1. Later in the work, neurotic analysands will generally come to realize the analyst only knows what they tell him. The transference love that arises here tends to be limited, when compared with the extreme love professed to and evinced by psychotics, and neurotics generally realize that their love for the analyst is produced by the situation and that it will most likely never be consummated in that situation. They may occasionally push the boundaries of the analytic frame, but rarely go to the extent seen in cases of psychosis.
2. The overriding, more global transference, as Lacan sees it, is that related to the subject-supposed-to-know. As an analysand, I feel able to pursue the exploration of the maze of my own bizarre thoughts and feelings because *the analyst holds the place of knowledge for me* when I myself feel terribly confused, anxious about my confusion, and despair of ever figuring anything out. The analyst remains calm in the face of obscurity, not knowing, and even nonsense, so I can too.

Transference has to do with a love of knowledge (not a desire to know or figure out), but it is of no help if it is just a worshiping of the person who we think has or possesses knowledge (we often find this sort of configuration when students fall in love with their professors, for example). The question for us in analysis is how to turn a patient who simply loves or worships someone who is knowledgeable into a patient who loves learning new things, discovering knowledge—in other words, how to inspire in the analysand a joy of deciphering the unconscious. It is not the same thing to *enjoy meaning*, which is usually provided by the analyst/professor, and to *enjoy deciphering*, which is done by the analysand (as encouraged and spurred on by the analyst).

3. An important point to note here is that what we don't see in psychotic transferences is both love and hate at the exact same time—this is what I call actual ambivalence—as we find in neurosis where one affect is conscious and the other is unconscious. As Freud puts it, "emotional ambivalence in the proper sense of the term ... is the simultaneous existence of love and hate towards the same object" (SE XIII, p. 157).

4. In erotomania we find alternating, extreme love for and hatred of the analyst, and/or the belief that the analyst has extreme love for and hatred of the analysand (Maleval, 2000, p. 449).

5. It was first used in the talk Lacan gave in Baltimore in 1966 at the structuralism conference, "Of Structure as an Inmixing of an Otherness Prerequisite to Any Subject Whatever," published in *The Structuralist Controversy* (Baltimore and London: Johns Hopkins University Press, 1970 [originally published in *Cahiers pour l'analyse*, 5, 1966, p. 70]), and then in his introduction to the French translation of Schreber's *Memoirs*. It was used again in Seminar XVI and then fairly often thereafter.

6. This reorientation of psychoanalytic work around jouissance retroactively affected the way many Lacanians worked with neurotics as well, but more on that another time.

7. Neurotics usually have far more social bonds, owing to the fact that, having undergone a highly significant loss (via separation and castration), they are always trying to get object *a* back from the Other. The psychotic, not having undergone such a loss, doesn't. That makes him, in Lacan's book, into a free man (*l'homme libre*): he has the object himself ("in his pocket," as Lacan puts it, although I would argue that object *a* cannot possibly function in the same way in psychosis as in neurosis due to the way it arises out of alienation and separation in neurosis). The psychotic isn't enslaved to trying to get it from the Other. He is not connected, bonded, glued, or tied to the Other by his quest for object *a*.

8. "Joyce le symptôme I" (Lacan, 1987, p. 21). But had he ever subscribed to it?
9. Bychowski (1996).
10. Conversations about their jouissance (as opposed to interpretations thereof) need not necessarily lead to a sex-change operation, the subject sometimes being content with simply cross dressing; but sometimes it may seem that the best thing to do is to support the subject's decision to get operated on (Maleval, 2019, p. 208). A French study from 1991 to 2009 at the Foch Hospital (in Suresnes) just outside of Paris showed that 95% of those who went through sex-change operations had no regret; 60% were satisfied, 25% unsatisfied, and 15% unsure. Most of those who were unsatisfied indicated that they did not like the aesthetics of the result, often feeling it was not convincing to others and thus their new social role was not easily accepted by others. Others were unhappy with the lack of functionality of the new sexual organ (p. 205).
11. The "death of the subject" in Schreber's terms.
12. Studies in different countries nevertheless suggest that the evolution of schizophrenia over time is favorable in 53 to 59% of cases.
13. The unidentified threat to the patient may lead her to suicide. Does a true delusion get constructed here? How can we help temper the self-destructive impulses? By gently calling into question the grounds for the self-accusation, perhaps. By helping locate the cause of the disturbance outside of the patient?
14. The man who killed Henri IV may well have been thinking along the same lines about the most beloved of the French kings.
15. Lacan once commented very simply that the real "is what is not going alright, what is blocking the wagon train [*charroi*], and even more so, what doesn't stop repetitively impeding its forward motion" (Lacan, 1975d, p. 183).
16. In the case of patients suffering bodily pains who receive a diagnosis of multiple sclerosis or fibromyalgia, the suffering itself may in some cases help define the body, give it limits and reality, and the diagnostic label may provide an explanation which is not *psychological* but rather genetic or hormonal.
17. See Fink 2014b, chapter 14.
18. An unexplained insistence, on the part of the head of the CMPS, that everyone show proof of Covid vaccinations and boosters (well after the end of the Covid insanity, and long after everyone else had stopped doing so) made it impossible for me to give this presentation on the scheduled date.

Chapter 3: The many faces of the imaginary

1. Lacan had perhaps read Lorenz's 1949 book, *Er redete mit dem Vieh, den Vögeln und den Fischen* (Vienna: Borotha-Schoeler), that was published in English in 1952 as *King Solomon's Ring*.
2. It could be tricky to take this analogy much further, insofar as many psychologists think of this bowing or bending over posture as defensive, involving protectiveness of one's soft fleshy abdomen area, whereas in many mammal species submissive postures involve exposing to one's potential attacker one's abdomen by lying on one's back, paws or legs in the air. This latter posture is associated, according to certain ethologists, with early relations between baby mammals and their mothers, the latter often licking their progeny's anal and genital regions in order to stimulate defecation and urination.
3. Colloquially, we might refer to this kind of facial expression as a "shit-eating grin."
4. Figure 3.5: happiness; Figure 3.6: anger; Figure 3.6: disgust. How many did you guess "correctly"?
5. Cf. Freud, SE VIII, p. 115, where the text is somewhat different: "What a liar you are!" broke out the other. "If you say you're going to Cracow, you want me to believe you're going to Lemberg. But I know that in fact you're going to Cracow. So why are you lying to me?"
6. Another possible example, which is mentioned by Darwin himself, is the way in which a certain patting of the paws on the part of cats, which apparently derives from their pushing on their mother's mammary glands during suckling when they are kittens, has become a kind of sign of pleasure itself, which appears when being scratched or caressed by their owners. Whether it is intended as a sign to someone else, whether another cat or a human being, is an open question.
7. As Freud (SE V, p. 511) put it, "To explain a thing means to trace it back to something already known" (see also SE XVI, p. 280).

Chapter 4: Love, warts and all

1. "*Vos symptômes à vous, c'est la seule chose qui, chez vous comme chez chacun, porte l'intérêt.*"
2. This paper was also given at Boston College on October 17, 2016, as part of an all-day conference entitled "Love and Mourning in the Constitution of the Subject: Recent Psychoanalytic Perspectives."

3. Cromwell was Lord Protector of England at the time. Lely had been portrait artist to Charles I and, following the restoration of the monarchy in 1660, was appointed as Charles II's "Principal Painter in Ordinary." Lely's painting style was, as was usual at the time, intended to flatter the sitter. Royalty in particular expected portraits to show them in the best possible light, if not to be outright fanciful.

    Cromwell did have a preference for being portrayed as a gentleman of military bearing, but was well-known to be opposed to all forms of personal vanity. It is plausible that he would have issued a "warts and all" instruction when being painted. Captain William Winde claimed Cromwell told Lely, "Mr Lely, I desire you would use all your skill to paint my picture truly like me, and not flatter me at all; but remark all these roughnesses, pimples, warts and everything as you see me, otherwise I will never pay a farthing for it."

4. "*Ce qui dans l'amour est aimé, c'est en effet ce qui est au-delà du sujet, c'est littéralement ce qu'il n'a pas.*" Consider Prince Charles's quip to his mother, Queen Elizabeth II, in the 2006 movie *The Queen*: "That was always the extraordinary thing about [Princess Diana]: her weaknesses and transgressions only made the public love her more."

5. As Lacan puts it in Seminar XX: "All love is based on a certain relationship between two unconscious knowledges" (p. 144).

6. "[*Ce qu'elle montre*] *dans cet amour exalté pour la dame, [c'est], comme nous le dit Freud, le modèle de l'amour absolument désintéressé, de l'amour pour rien.* […] *Ce qu'elle lui démontre, c'est comment on peut aimer quelqu'un, non pas seulement pour ce qu'il a, mais littéralement pour ce qu'il n'a pas.*" On this point, see Fink, 2004, p. 18.

7. Lacan proffers this formulation a few years later: "*Elle se fait amant. En d'autres termes, elle se pose dans ce qu'elle n'a pas, le phallus, et pour bien montrer qu'elle l'a, elle le donne. C'est en effet une façon tout à fait démonstrative. Elle se comporte, nous dit Freud, vis-à-vis de la Dame avec un grand D, comme un cavalier servant, comme un homme, comme celui qui peut lui sacrifier ce qu'il a, son phallus*" (Seminar X, class given on January 23, 1963; see, also, Seminar VI, p. 549).

8. It was not Ernst Lanzer, as Patrick Mahony would have us believe.

9. Betty Joseph (1985) even goes so far as to suggest that a whole group of people (in a graduate seminar in which they were discussing a case) felt a pressure to "understand at all costs" that had been projected into the therapist recounting the case by her patient (p. 448).

10. For a detailed critique of the concept of projective identification, see Fink, 2007, chapter 7.
11. Renik (1993) even goes so far as to say that "The term interpretation dates from a conception of the psychoanalytic process that is now generally criticized," as if he, like certain others, were announcing the end of interpretation (p. 413).
12. Blanton (1971) also claims that by 1935, Freud had "learned the difficult art of countertransference. He gives of himself—but not indiscriminately or in a way that would burden the patient with the necessity of returning affection for affection, of like for like" (pp. 64–65).

Chapter 5: Notions of love in Lacan's later work

1. Lacan's image here is perhaps not unrelated to one Ovid provides, with which Lacan was undoubtedly familiar: "Now having seen Narcissus, she [Echo] was struck by his beauty, enamored, followed along behind him, going from bush to bush, eager for yet a closer look at this marvelous creature. The closer she came, the more ardently she burned, as a torch with its coating of sulfur will burst into flames from another torch that is held nearby" (*Metamorphoses*, III:372–378).
2. Lacan, 1968, p. 46; cf. Allouch, 2009, p. 448.
3. Allouch (2009, pp. 408, 454) associates this with Aristotle's notion, in his logic, that it is more worthy to be loved by one's beloved than to be granted his sexual favors; in this sense the lover burns slowly instead of being quickly consumed. This might be thought to characterize what Socrates does: he burns with desire for Alcibiades but never consummates the relationship.
4. Instead of "well-meaning neutrality," Freud talks about "sympathetic understanding," *Einfühlung* (SE XII, p. 140).
5. "*Il n'y a d'amour que d'un nom, comme chacun le sait d'expérience, et le moment où le nom est prononcé, de celui ou de celle à qui s'adresse notre amour, nous savons très bien que c'est un seuil qui a la plus grande importance*" (Lacan, Seminar X, class given on July 3, 1963).
6. See Allouch, 2009, pp. 403ff.
7. "*Qui n'est pas amoureux de son inconscient erre*" [...] *Il n'y a pas besoin de se savoir amoureux de son inconscient pour ne pas errer, il n'y a qu'à se laisser faire, en être la dupe. Pour la première fois dans l'histoire, il vous est possible, à vous d'errer, c'est-à-dire de refuser d'aimer votre inconscient, puisque enfin*

vous savez ce que c'est: un savoir, un savoir emmerdant" (Seminar XXI, class given on June 11, 1974).

"Whoever is not in love with his unconscious goes astray, etc." When we allow ourselves to *errer*, to go astray, the unconscious allows us to reach the "pure real," instead of the "scant reality" we deal with usually—that of fantasy. Hence the extreme importance of love for the unconscious.

8. What is loved in analysis is not so much knowledge itself as the subject-supposed-to-know (Allouch, 2009, p. 412)—that is, the fantasy that *someone* is all-knowing.
9. "She runs away from me since I could tell her the last word of the secret of her illness."
10. According to Allouch (2009, p. 437), S_2, in any case, stands, at this point in Lacan's work, not for knowledge but for double meanings (or for a meaning doubled by its sound). He is referring there to Seminar XXIV (class given on March 15, 1977). In the same class, Lacan talks about "dissolving symptoms" by "intervening symbolically." In Seminar XXV (class given on November 15, 1977), he refers to "undoing [*défaire*]" symptoms "through speech."
11. Note that FOS sounds just like *fosse* (ditch), which is not a very pretty word in French, being part of *fosse septique* (septic tank) and *fosse commune* (mass grave). See Seminar XXII, class given on January 14, 1975.
12. There is also the idea here of a one that talks all by itself, never being able to reach another; S_1 doesn't ultimately reach S_2 and lovers don't ultimately reach each other. Ultimate knowledge (S_2) is never reached. The partner's "being" is never reached.
13. It is not a sort of direct "communication of unconsciouses," the kind Freud postulated in "The Unconscious": "the unconscious of one human being can react upon that of another" (SE XIV, p. 194).
14. To Lacan, the injunction to love thy neighbor as thyself means the abolition of sexual difference, the total setting aside of sexual difference when it comes to Christian love (Seminar XXI, class given on December 18, 1973).
15. He says he was convinced of this by reading a biography of *Queen Victoria* written by Lytton Strachey.

A few of the notions in this paper were also presented on October 14, 2017, in Portland to the Oregon Psychoanalytic Center, and again on October 28, 2017, in Manhattan to the Center for Modern Psychoanalytic Studies.

Chapter 6: Why people aren't what they seem to be, or what Freud teaches us about repression

1. If you have ever wrestled with a dog that you know very well, you may have noticed something similar when the dog begins to growl at you when the wrestling gets a bit tough, but then instead sneezes. It is as if the dog suppresses an aggressive impulse to bite you and then does something related and yet unrelated with its mouth.
2. Consider the case of the character played by Meg Ryan in *French Kiss*.
3. They sometimes also involve sexual feelings toward a parent or close relative, and simultaneous moral repulsion at such feelings.

Chapter 7: The slings and arrows of outrageous fortune

1. Intersecting the theme of lying that I return to later, it is interesting to note that all of the money that J inherited came from illegal business dealings that his father conducted alongside his legal business. His father, too, apparently lied a great deal.
2. St. Damien died of leprosy he contracted by working with lepers. This may be related to psoriatic "stigmata" on J's hands and feet.
3. Although J jumped to the conclusion that his father felt guilty about what he had done to his son, his father was actually talking about feeling guilty toward his own father: he had begrudgingly worked in his father's business and ostensibly felt guilty for not having wanted to.
4. They were obviously miles from suspecting his guilt might have something to do with giving up on his own desire.
5. This common expression is a paraphrase of William Blake's 1810 poem "The Liar":

Deceiver, dissembler
Your trousers are alight
From what pole or gallows
Shall they dangle in the night?

When I asked of your career
Why did you have to kick my rear
With that stinking lie of thine
Proclaiming that you owned a mine?

When you asked to borrow my stallion
To visit a nearby moored galleon

How could I ever know that you
Intended to turn him into glue?

What red devil of mendacity
Grips your soul with such tenacity?
Will one you cruelly shower with lies
Put a pistol ball between your eyes?

What internal serpent
Has lent you his forked tongue?
From what pit of foul deceit
Are all these whoppers sprung?

Deceiver, dissembler
Your trousers are alight
From what pole or gallows
Do they dangle in the night?

6. Strangely enough, J's grades suddenly fell at that point, he having been a fairly good student prior to that; as if he was suddenly doing worse when his father was doing better.
7. "This confirms what I told you was essential to the mainspring of comedy, which is always, in the end, a reference to the phallus" (Seminar VIII, p. 94).
8. He also characterized sexual intercourse as a way of saying "fuck you" to his mother; it is matricide (although he said "marricide"): killing his mother as well as killing marriage as an institution. To not be able to have it, then, is not to commit matricide.
9. This formulation has a decidedly Orwellian ring to it; see also "The Freud Man and the Fundamental Fantasy" in Fink, 2014b, pp. 210–214.
10. He didn't ask himself whether *anything* could ever serve as absolute proof of unconditional love. He inevitably ended up acting so abominably as to chase every woman away (he often could not even respect them when they did sometimes put up with his horrible treatment of them).
11. Freud (1910), "A Special Type of Choice of Object Made by Men," *SE* XI, p. 166. See my in-depth discussion of this point in *Lacan on Love*, pp. 9–11.

   J said he felt constant competition with his father regarding women; for example, he wanted his father to be blown away by his college girlfriend's good looks so that the father would then go nuts for her and pine for her (he didn't and J was quite disappointed about this). He once even said he felt all women were his father's; to have one for himself was thus to take her from him.

12. He once said that he felt like he was sucking every man's dick (not just those of psychiatrists), whoring for men, acting the part of their "bitches."
13. J seemed to need to feel his father was angered by all of his jouissance; in particular, his anger at J's masturbation would prove he was angered by J's jouissance of mom, confirming that J was a genuine, formidable rival in his father's eyes.
14. Would psychoanalysis be able to or want to dominate him? This was his challenge to me and to the field as a whole.
15. The context in which he said this made it ambiguous as to whether he was referring to his penis or psychoanalysis (he felt that if his penis worked he wouldn't need me anymore).
16. Another patient contemplated "what I could do on my own to be a healthy person," as opposed to a victim (Whitaker, 2010, p. 171).
17. His worst and most tenacious skin conditions were on his face and back. Note that his mother's favorite football team was the Washington Redskins.

    Certain skin problems cleared up easily, one in particular—psoriasis on his hands and feet—after ashamedly repeating to me a racist joke his father used to tell about why black people have white hands and feet, the purported reason for which was that the sun never shined on them when they were climbing around in the trees (as if they were monkeys). The day after he recounted the joke—after having told me about other racist comments his father would make—the psoriasis on his hands and feet went away.

    J once indicated that his skin problems began shortly after his college girlfriend (who might well be characterized as "the love of his life") broke up with him.
18. As a side note, let me indicate that it took J a full three years to wean himself from the psychotropic medications he was taking and that he complained of having every withdrawal symptom under the sun, many of which were clearly suggested to him by online forums he found where people complained about these medications. Reading their complaints, he would suddenly realize he was having the exact same withdrawal symptoms as they were. Curiously enough, he never

complained, the whole time he was taking the full prescribed doses of these medications, of having any of *their* well-known or not so well-known side effects (apart from suppressed libido). In other words, it seemed consonant with his self-image as someone who was sick to need medications, but it bothered him to be losing that self-image as he cut back; and he therefore blamed every little sensation in his body and any fatigue or unpleasant mood on withdrawal effects. This is not to say that there are no such well-documented effects, but, given the excruciatingly slow rate at which J reduced the dosage of medications he was taking, my impression was that most of the sensations and states he complained of were more likely due to smoking pot, alcohol-related hangovers, or other activities than to withdrawal from psychotropic medications.

19. Were we to try to formulate J's fundamental fantasy as Freud formulates fantasies in "A Child is Being Beaten," we might propose the following:
    1) I am being seduced by my mother (my father witnesses this).
    2) I am being molested/beaten/dominated by my father (because of the seduction).
    3) A girl is being molested (by a dirty old man); or: everyone wants to molest me (as a young girl).
    Cf. "The Freud Man and the Fundamental Fantasy" in Fink, 2014b.

Chapter 8: What makes translating Lacan's work so difficult

1. This doesn't stop him from occasionally rereading and admiring work he'd done in the past (see, for example, Seminar XVIII, chapters 6–7).
2. Here he is no doubt echoing Cheng Yi's dictum, "The Sage's word is transformed in relation to the person to whom it is addressed" (cited in Jullien, 2000, p. 277).
3. The new *Écrits: A Selection* that came out in 2002 has thus far sold about 17,000 copies.
4. See my comments on smoldering in Chapter 5 in this volume.
5. This paper was also delivered as a keynote at the 2018 Lacan *Écrits* Conference held in Ghent, Belgium, on September 21–22, 2018. It appeared in Spanish in *Saltos: Training, Research and Transmission of Psychoanalysis*, 7 (2021), and will appear in Italian in Antonio Di Ciaccia's journal *La psicoanalisi*.

Chapter 9: Lacan in "translation"

1. *Tige* means stem (of a plant) and the translation "to graft" would have been creative, albeit incorrect.
2. Of course, sometimes it is better not to try to understand too much, and to simply translate as best one can and let others puzzle it out. In this case, "over there" (instead of "down there") would have at least allowed readers to try to figure out where "over there" was.
3. Here is the revised version included in *Écrits*, p. 727: "After that, the reality principle loses the discordance that supposedly characterizes it in Freud's work when, on the basis of a comparison of texts, it is thought to be split between a notion of reality that includes psychical reality and another that makes it the correlate of the perception-consciousness system."
4. Sheridan would seem to be asking us to believe that Lacan simply wants us to move on in the discussion at hand ("On to the phantasy …") or that the graph inscribes something on (to) fantasy. While the latter possibility is incorrect, it is at least plausible.
5. The rest of the sentence confirms this reading: "The graph shows that desire adjusts to [or: takes its cue from] fantasy as posited in this way—like the ego does in relation to the body image—but the graph also shows the inversion of the misrecognitions on which the one and the other are based, respectively." Note that on Graph 3 in "Subversion of the Subject," desire (d) and fantasy ($\$ \lozenge a$) are located at the same vertical level (one adapting or adjusting to the other), with the former on the right and the latter on the left; lower down, the ego (m) is on the left and the body image, $i(a)$, is on the right. This seems to be the "inversion" Lacan is referring to here.
6. For related discussions of the dream, see Soler, 1996, and Fink, 2004 (chapter 1); 1997 (pp. 125–127).
7. For an extensive discussion of this point see Fink, 2004 (chapter 3).
8. See Fink, 2004 (chapter 1).
9. University of Minnesota Press balked at my plan to include this paper in *Lacan to the Letter* (2004), as did Routledge in my two-volume collection entitled *Against Understanding* (2014), but Dany Nobus was, fortunately, willing to publish it in his short-lived *Journal for Lacanian Studies*, 2, 2 (2004): 264–281.

Chapter 10: The emphasis on the unconscious is back

1. Lacan even says that he is trying to forge a *folisophie* (Seminar XXIII, p. 128), combining *folie* (folly or madness) with philosophy! And at a press conference held in Rome on October 29, 1974, he said, "I don't create any sort of philosophy—on the contrary, I distrust philosophy like the plague" (Lacan, 1975c, p. 26).
2. See Maleval, 2019.
3. I was not aware, at the time of the interview, of Domenico Cosenza's fine book entitled *Le refus dans l'anorexie* (Rennes, France: Presses Universitaires de Rennes, 2014).

Chapter 14: Introduction to Seminar VI

1. Seminar XVI came out in 2024, and Seminar XVIII should be out in 2025.
2. Let me point out two minor errors I found while rereading Seminar VI for the book launch today:
   1) On p. 117, the prime on a' in the upper righthand corner of the L Schema is missing.
   2) On p. 381, ten lines from the bottom: change "itself" to "himself."

Chapter 15: Brief remarks made at the 25th anniversary of A Clinical Introduction to Lacanian Psychoanalysis

1. Comments were made by Yael Baldwin, Stephanie Swales, Cristina Laurita, Kristen Hennessy, Celeste Pietrusza, and Diana Cuello.
2. They are discussed at length in Chapter 2 of the present collection.

Chapter 16: Review of Elisabeth Roudinesco's biography entitled Jacques Lacan (New York: Columbia University Press, 1997)

1. I should know: I was asked to help out and spent weeks correcting the references and notes!

Chapter 17: A few notes on supervision

1. Certain Lacanians view it that way and sometimes even use scansion during supervision, clearly suggesting to their supervisees that supervision is a continuation of their analyses.

2. Obviously, if you believe analysis is all about the transference/countertransference, you'll end up focusing on that in supervision and worry about enactments and repetitions on the part of supervisee and supervisor of what is going on in the analysis. If, however, you believe analysis is about something else, you'll center your work on something else.
3. For a Lacanian perspective, see Dulsster, Vanheule, Hermans, and Hennissen, 2021.
4. For further considerations on self-disclosure, see the end of "Love, Warts and All" in Chapter 4 of this collection.

BIBLIOGRAPHY

Lacan, J. (1953–1977). The Seminars cited here in order:

1. *The Seminar of Jacques Lacan, Book I: Freud's Papers on Technique (1953–1954)*. J.-A. Miller (Ed.), J. Forrester (Trans.). New York: W. W. Norton, 1988.
3. *The Seminar of Jacques Lacan, Book III: The Psychoses (1955–1956)*. J.-A. Miller (Ed.), R. Grigg (Trans.). New York: W. W. Norton, 1993.
4. *Le séminaire, Livre IV: La relation d'objet*. Paris: Seuil, 1994.
6. *The Seminar of Jacques Lacan, Book VI: Desire and Its Interpretation (1958–1959)*. J.-A. Miller, B. Fink (Trans.). Cambridge: Polity, 2019.
7. *The Seminar of Jacques Lacan, Book VII: The Ethics of Psychoanalysis (1959–1960)*. J.-A. Miller (Ed.), D. Porter (Trans.). New York: W. W. Norton, 1992.
8. *The Seminar of Jacques Lacan, Book VIII: Transference (1960–1961)*. J.-A. Miller (Ed.), B. Fink (Trans.). Cambridge: Polity, 2015.
9. *Le séminaire, Livre IX: L'identification* (1961–1962). (Unpublished).
10. *Le séminaire, Livre X: L'angoisse*. Paris: Seuil, 2004.
11. *Le séminaire, Livre XI: Les quatre concepts fondamentaux de la psychanalyse*. Paris: Seuil, 1973. *The Seminar of Jacques Lacan, Book XI: The Four Fundamental Concepts of Psychoanalysis*. J.-A. Miller (Ed.), A. Sheridan (Trans.). New York: W. W. Norton, 1978a.

13 *Le séminaire, Livre XIII: L'objet de la psychanalyse* (1965–1966). (Unpublished).
14 *Le séminaire, Livre XIV: La logique du fantasme*. Paris: Seuil, 2023.
16 *The Seminar of Jacques Lacan, Book XVI: From an Other to the other (1968–1969)*. J.-A. Miller (Ed.), B. Fink (Trans.). Cambridge: Polity, 2024.
18 *Le séminaire, Livre XVIII, D'un discours qui ne serait pas du semblant (1970–1971)*. J.-A. Miller (Ed.). Paris: Seuil, 2007.
20 *Le séminaire, Livre XX: Encore*. Paris: Seuil, 1975b. *The Seminar of Jacques Lacan, Book XX: Encore (1972–1973)*. J.-A. Miller (Ed.), B. Fink (Trans.). New York: W. W. Norton, 1998.
21 *Le séminaire, Livre XXI: Les non dupes errent* (1973–1974). (Unpublished).
22 *Le séminaire, Livre XXII: RSI* (1974–1975). (Unpublished).
23 *Le séminaire, Livre XXIII: Le sinthome*. Paris: Seuil, 2005.
24 *Le séminaire, Livre XXIV: L'insu que sait de l'une-bévue s'aile à mourre* (1976–1977). (Unpublished).
25 *Le séminaire, Livre XXV: Le moment de conclure* (1977). (Unpublished).

REFERENCES

Allouch, J. (2009). *L'amour Lacan*. Paris: EPEL.
Avital, E., & Jablonka, E. (2000). *Animal Traditions: Behavioural Inheritance in Evolution*. Cambridge: Cambridge University Press.
Baldwin, Y. (2015). *Let's Keep Talking: Lacanian Tales of Love, Sex, and other Catastrophes*. London: Karnac.
Beaussant, P. (2002). *Forqueray, Pièces de viole*. CD by Jordi Savall.
Blanton, M. G. (1971). *Diary of my Analysis with Sigmund Freud*. New York: Hawthorn.
Bollas, C. (1983). Expressive uses of the countertransference. *Contemporary Psychoanalysis, 19*: 1–34.
Bowie, M. (1991). *Lacan*. Cambridge, MA: Harvard University Press.
Bychowski, G. (1996). Psychosis precipitated by psychoanalysis. *Psychoanalytic Quarterly, 35*(3): 327–339.
Cervantes Saavedra, M. de (1995). *The History of that Ingenious Gentleman, Don Quijote de la Mancha*. B. Raffel (Trans.). New York: W. W. Norton.
Chauvin, R. (1941). Contribution à l'étude physiologique du Criquet pélerin et du déterminisme des phénomènes grégaires [Contribution to the physiological study of grasshoppers and the determination of gregarious traits]. *Annales de la Société entomologique de France, 1*: 1–137; 3: 133–272.

Cosenza, D. (2014). *Le refus dans l'anorexie*. Rennes, France: Presses Universitaires de Rennes.
Darwin, C. (1872). *The Expression of the Emotions in Man and Animals*. New York: D. Appleton, 1899.
de Waal, F. B. M., & Tyack, P. L. (Eds.) (2003). *Animal Social Complexity: Intelligence, Culture, and Individualized Societies*. Cambridge, MA: Harvard University Press.
Dryden, J. (1992). On translation. In: R. Schulte & J. Biguenet (Eds.), *Theories of Translation: An Anthology of Essays from Dryden to Derrida* (pp. 17–31). Chicago, IL: University of Chicago Press.
Dulsster, D., Vanheule, S., Hermans, G., & Hennissen, V. (2021). Supervision from a Lacanian Perspective Considered Closely: A Qualitative Study. *British Journal of Psychotherapy, 37*(2): 1–21.
ECF, collective (1997a). *La conversation d'Arcachon: Cas rares, les inclassables de la clinique*. Paris: Agalma-Seuil.
ECF, collective (1997b). *Le conciliabule d'Angers*. Paris: Agalma-Seuil.
ECF, collective (2005). *La psychose ordinaire: La convention d'Antibes*. Paris: Agalma-Seuil.
Falzeder, E. (1994). My grand-patient, my chief tormentor: A hitherto unnoticed case of Freud's and the consequences. *Psychoanalytic Quarterly, 63*: 297–331.
Fink, B. (1997). *A Clinical Introduction to Lacan: Theory and Technique*. Cambridge, MA: Harvard University Press.
Fink, B. (2004). *Lacan to the Letter: Reading Écrits Closely*. Minneapolis, MN: University of Minnesota Press.
Fink, B. (2007). *Fundamentals of Psychoanalytic Technique: A Lacanian Approach for Practitioners*. New York: W. W. Norton.
Fink, B. (2014a). *Against Understanding: Vol. 1. Commentary and Critique in a Lacanian Key*. London: Routledge.
Fink, B. (2014b). *Against Understanding: Vol. 2. Cases and Commentary in a Lacanian Key*. London: Routledge.
Fink, B. (2016). *Lacan on Love: An Exploration of Lacan's Seminar VIII*, Transference. Cambridge: Polity.
Fink, B. (2017). *A Clinical Introduction to Freud: Techniques for Everyday Practice*. New York: W. W. Norton.
Freud, S. (1953–1974). *The Standard Edition of the Complete Psychological Works of Sigmund Freud* (Vols. I–XXIV). London: Hogarth.
Freud, S. (2000). *L'homme aux rats*. Paris: Presses Universitaires de France.
Gherovici, P. (2003). *The Puerto Rican Syndrome*. New York: Other Press.
Grosskurth, P. (1987). *Melanie Klein: Her World and Her Work*. Cambridge, MA: Harvard University Press.

Joseph, B. (1985). Transference: The total situation. *International Journal of Psychoanalysis, 66*: 447–454.
Jullien, F. (2000). *Detour and Access: Strategies of Meaning in China and Greece*. S. Hawkes (Trans.). New York: Zone.
Kardiner, A. (1977). *My Analysis with Freud: Reminiscences*. New York: W. W. Norton.
Khoury, M. (2006). Une séance à mille temps (A thousand different session lengths). *Revue française de psychanalyse, 70*(1): 83–106.
Kuhn, T. S. (1962). *The Structure of Scientific Revolutions*. Chicago, IL: University of Chicago Press.
Lacan, J. (1932). *De la psychose paranoïaque dans ses rapports avec la personnalité* (The relationship between paranoiac psychosis and personality). Paris: Seuil, 1980.
Lacan, J. (1953). Some reflections on the ego. *International Journal of Psychoanalysis, 34*(1): 11–17.
Lacan, J. (1961–1962). *Le séminaire, Livre IX: L'identification*. (Unpublished).
Lacan, J. (1965–1966). *Le séminaire, Livre XIII: L'objet de la psychanalyse*. (Unpublished).
Lacan, J. (1966). *Écrits*. Paris: Seuil.
Lacan, J. (1967). Petit discours aux psychiatres. (Lecture given on November 10, 1967; unpublished.)
Lacan, J. (1968). De Rome 53 à Rome 67: La psychanalyse. Raison d'un échec. *Scilicet, 1*: 42–50.
Lacan, J. (1970). Of structure as an inmixing of an otherness prerequisite to any subject whatever. In: R. A. Macksey (Ed.), *The Structuralist Controversy*. Baltimore, MD: Johns Hopkins University Press.
Lacan, J. (1972). Seminar on "The Purloined Letter." *Yale French Studies, 48*: 39–72. J. Mehlman (Trans.). (Reprinted in: J. Muller & W. Richardson (Eds.), *The Purloined Poe*. Baltimore, MD: Johns Hopkins University Press, 1988.)
Lacan, J. (1973). *Le séminaire, Livre XI: Les quatre concepts fondamentaux de la psychanalyse*. Paris: Seuil.
Lacan, J. (1973–1974). *Le séminaire, Livre XXI: Les non dupes errent*. (Unpublished).
Lacan, J. (1974). *Télévision*. Paris: Seuil.
Lacan, J. (1974–1975). *Le séminaire, Livre XXII: RSI*. (Unpublished).
Lacan, J. (1975a). Introduction à l'édition allemande d'un premier volume des *Écrits* (Introduction to the first volume of *Écrits* in German). *Scilicet, 5*: 11–17.
Lacan, J. (1975b). *Le séminaire, Livre XX: Encore*. Paris: Seuil.
Lacan, J. (1975c). Press conference held in Rome on October 29, 1974. *Lettres de l'École freudienne, 16*: 6–26.

Lacan, J. (1975d). La troisième. *Lettres de l'École freudienne, 16*: 177–203.
Lacan, J. (1976–1977). *Le séminaire, Livre XXIV: L'insu que sait de l'une-bévue s'aile à mourre*. (Unpublished).
Lacan, J. (1977). *Écrits: A Selection*. A. Sheridan (Trans.). New York: W. W. Norton.
Lacan, J. (1978a). *The Seminar of Jacques Lacan, Book XI: The Four Fundamental Concepts of Psychoanalysis*. J.-A. Miller (Ed.), A. Sheridan (Trans.). New York: W. W. Norton.
Lacan, J. (1978b). L'expérience de la passe. *Lettres de l'École, 23*: 180–181.
Lacan, J. (1981). Intervention de Jacques Lacan à Bruxelles. *Quarto* (Supplément belge à *La lettre mensuelle de l'École de la cause freudienne*), 2.
Lacan, J. (1982). *Feminine Sexuality: Jacques Lacan and the École freudienne*. New York: W. W. Norton.
Lacan, J. (1986). Conférence de Bruxelles sur l'éthique de la psychanalyse (lecture given on September 3, 1960). *La Revue Belge de Psychanalyse, 4*: 163–187.
Lacan, J. (1987). *Joyce avec Lacan*. Paris: Navarin.
Lacan, J. (1988). *The Seminar of Jacques Lacan, Book I: Freud's Papers on Technique (1953–1954)*. J.-A. Miller (Ed.), J. Forrester (Trans.). New York: W. W. Norton.
Lacan, J. (1989a). Kant with Sade. J. B. Swenson (Trans.). *October, 51*: 55–75.
Lacan, J. (1989b). Science and truth. B. Fink (Trans.). *Newsletter of the Freudian Field, 3*(1/2): 4–29.
Lacan, J. (1990). *Television: A Challenge to the Psychoanalytic Establishment*. D. Hollier, R. Krauss, & A. Michelson (Trans.). New York: W. W. Norton.
Lacan, J. (1992). *The Seminar of Jacques Lacan, Book VII: The Ethics of Psychoanalysis (1959–1960)*. J.-A. Miller (Ed.), D. Porter (Trans.). New York: W. W. Norton.
Lacan, J. (1993). *The Seminar of Jacques Lacan, Book III: The Psychoses (1955–1956)*. J.-A. Miller (Ed.), R. Grigg (Trans.). New York: W. W. Norton.
Lacan, J. (1994). *Le séminaire, Livre IV: La relation d'objet*. Paris: Seuil.
Lacan, J. (1998). *The Seminar of Jacques Lacan, Book XX: Encore (1972–1973)*. J.-A. Miller (Ed.), B. Fink (Trans.). New York: W. W. Norton.
Lacan, J. (2001). *Autres Écrits*. Paris: Seuil.
Lacan, J. (2004). *Le séminaire, Livre X: L'angoisse*. Paris: Seuil.
Lacan, J. (2005). *Le séminaire, Livre XXIII: Le sinthome*. Paris: Seuil.
Lacan, J. (2006). *Écrits: The First Complete Edition in English*. B. Fink (Trans.). New York: W. W. Norton. (Original work published 1966.)
Lacan, J. (2007). *Le séminaire, Livre XVIII, D'un discours qui ne serait pas du semblant (1970–1971)*. J.-A. Miller (Ed.). Paris: Seuil.
Lacan, J. (2013). *On the Names-of-the-Father*. J.-A. Miller (Ed.), B. Fink (Trans.). Cambridge: Polity.

Lacan, J. (2015). *The Seminar of Jacques Lacan, Book VIII: Transference (1960–1961)*. J.-A. Miller (Ed.), B. Fink (Trans.). Cambridge: Polity.
Lacan, J. (2019). *The Seminar of Jacques Lacan, Book VI: Desire and Its Interpretation (1958–1959)*. J.-A. Miller (Ed.), B. Fink (Trans.). Cambridge: Polity.
Lacan, J. (2024). *The Seminar of Jacques Lacan, Book XVI: From an Other to the other (1968–1969)*. J.-A. Miller (Ed.), B. Fink (Trans.). Cambridge: Polity.
Little, M. (1990). *Psychotic Anxieties and Containment: A Personal Record of an Analysis with Winnicott*. Northvale, NJ: Jason Aronson.
Lorenz, C. (1949). *Er redete mit dem Vieh, den Vögeln und den Fischen*. Vienna: Borotha-Schoeler.
Malan, D. H. (1995). *Individual Psychotherapy and the Science of Psychodynamics*. London: Arnold.
Maleval, J.-C. (2000). *La forclusion du nom-du-père: Le concept et sa clinique*. Paris: Seuil.
Maleval, J.-C. (2011). *Logique du délire*. Rennes, France: Presses Universitaires de Rennes.
Maleval, J.-C. (2019). *Repères pour la psychose ordinaire*. Paris: Navarin.
Matthews, L. H. (1939). Visual stimulation and ovulation in pigeons. *Proceedings of the Royal Society*, Series B, 126: 557–560.
Miller, J.-A. (2003). Contre-transfert et intersubjectivité. *La cause freudienne*, 53: 7–39.
Miller, M. (2011). *Lacanian Psychotherapy: Theory and Practical Applications*. London: Routledge.
Ogden, T. H. (1994). The analytic third: Working with intersubjective clinical facts. In: S. A. Mitchell & L. Aron (Eds.), *Relational Psychoanalysis: The Emergence of a Tradition*. Hillsdale, NJ: Analytic Press, 1999.
Ovid (c. AD 8). *Metamorphoses*. R. Humphries (Trans.). Bloomington, IN: Indiana University Press, 2018.
Peoc'h, M. (2022). *Solutions élégantes à la psychose: Une clinique lacanienne auprès des sujets psychotiques*. Rennes, France: Presses Universitaires de Rennes.
Pommier, G. (1996). *Le dénouement d'une analyse*. Paris: Flammarion.
Renik, O. (1993). Analytic interaction: Conceptualizing technique in light of the analyst's irreducible subjectivity. In: S. A. Mitchell & L. Aron (Eds.), *Relational Psychoanalysis: The Emergence of a Tradition*. Hillsdale, NJ: Analytic Press, 1999.
Roudinesco, E. (1990). *Jacques Lacan & Co.: A History of Psychoanalysis in France 1925–1985*. J. Mehlman (Trans.). Chicago, IL: University of Chicago Press.
Roudinesco, E. (1997). *Jacques Lacan*. New York: Columbia University Press.
Schleiermacher, F. (1992). On the different methods of translating. In: R. Schulte & J. Biguenet (Eds.), *Theories of Translation: An Anthology*

of Essays from Dryden to Derrida (pp. 36–54). Chicago, IL: University of Chicago Press.

Schreber, D. P. (1988). *Memoirs of My Nervous Illness*. Cambridge, MA: Harvard University Press.

Sokal, A., & Bricmont, J. (1998). *Fashionable Nonsense: Postmodern Intellectuals' Abuse of Science* [British title: *Intellectual Impostures*]. New York: Picador.

Soler, C. (1990). Le sujet psychotique dans la psychanalyse. In: *Psychose et creation: Actualité de l'école anglaise*. Paris: GRAPP.

Soler, C. (1996). Hysteria and Obsession. In: R. Feldstein, B. Fink, & M. Jaanus (Eds.), *Reading Seminars I and II: Lacan's Return to Freud*. Albany, NY: SUNY Press.

Soler, C. (2003). *Ce que Lacan disait des femmes*. Paris: Éditions du Champ lacanien. (In English, see Soler, C. [2006]. *What Lacan Said about Women*. New York: Other Press.)

Soler, C. (2015). *Lacanian Affects: The Function of Affect in Lacan's Work*. B. Fink (Trans.). London: Routledge.

Spoto, D. (1993). *Marilyn Monroe: The Biography*. New York: HarperCollins.

Swales, S. S. (2012). *Perversion: A Lacanian Psychoanalytic Approach to the Subject*. London: Routledge.

Sylvestre, M. (1987). *Demain la psychanalyse*. Paris: Navarin.

Thorpe, W. H. (1979). *Origins and Rise of Ethology: The Science of the Natural Behaviour of Animals*. London: Heinemann Educational Books/Praeger.

Weinstein, L., Winer, J., & Ornstein, E. (2009). Supervision and self-disclosure: Modes of supervisory interaction. *Journal of the American Psychoanalytic Association, 57*: 1379–1400.

Whitaker, R. (2010). *The Anatomy of an Epidemic: Magic Bullets, Psychiatric Drugs, and the Astonishing Rise of Mental Illness in America*. New York: Crown.

Winnicott, D. W. (1958a). Metapsychological and clinical aspects of regression within the psycho-analytical set-up. In: *Collected Papers: Through Pediatrics to Psycho-Analysis* (pp. 278–294). London: Tavistock.

Winnicott, D. W. (1958b). Clinical varieties of transference. In: *Collected Papers: Through Pediatrics to Psycho-Analysis* (pp. 295–299). London: Tavistock.

INDEX

affect, 9, 145
   anxiety, 10
   displacement of, 158
   ethical perspective on, 11–12
   hunting, 9
   integrating thought and, 10
   moral failing, 11
   Rat Man's guilty, 111, 167–168
affections, overemphasized, 146.
      See also deception
Allouch, J., 126, 127, 139
analyst(s), 303
   -analysand relationship, 12–13, 43
   contemporary analysts, 10
   desires for affection and
      recognition, 121–122
   disinclination, 117
   paradox of analyst's role, 122
   role, 10–11, 12, 13
   self-disclosure, 120–121
analytic
   setting, 12, 25
   third, 118–119

"anchoring point," 31
animal behavior, 308
   deception and intentionality, 88
   feigning and symbolism, 88–89
   imaginary in, 77–79
   signs and social interactions, 91
   smiling, 81
   symbolic behavior and number
      sense, 91–92
anxiety, 10, 144–145. *See also* deception
   separation, 15–16
Aristophanes' myth, 133–134
"as if" personality, 55
"ataraxia," 128
attraction in human beings, 79
automatic thinking. *See* "mental
      automatism"
Avital, E., 78, 88

Bailly, L., 35
Baldwin, Y., 33, 317
bared-teeth grin, 81–82
Beaussant, P., 214

"bedrock of castration," 17–18
Bernardi, R., 32–35
Blake, W., 312
Blanton, M. G., 310
body language, 303
Bollas, C., 119
Borromean knot, 287
Bowie, M., 229
Bricmont, J., 217
"bungled actions," 149
"button tie," 31

castrating function. See "paternal function"
castration, 18
Chauvin, R., 77
"choice, forced," 20
"clinic," 282
Clinical Introduction to Freud, A, 271–276
Clinical Introduction to Lacanian Psychoanalysis, A, 281–282, 317
"compromise formations," 53
conscious, 148–151
contemporary analysts, 10. See also analyst(s)
Cosenza, D., 317
couch, 25–27, 299
countertransference, 7–9
  dismantling myth of transference, 8
  hate, 110
  intuition, 8–9
  love, 110
  and projection of responsibility, 114
  reframing, 115–116
  use and abuse of, 110–122
"crazy love," 11, 133–135
Cromwell, O., 105, 309

Darwin, C., 80–82, 308
deception, 143, 162, 312
  anxiety as mask, 144–145
  common occurrences, 144–147
  conscious and unconscious, 148–151
  disingenuous praise, 146
  excessive excuses, 145
  Freudian analysis of conflict and neurosis, 155–156
  hidden self in moments of uninhibited expression, 145
  intricacies of opposites, 147–148
  love and hate in dreams, 146
  overemphasized affections, 146
  projection in relationships, 144
  psychological defense mechanisms, 151–154
  repression, 151–154, 158–162
  unconscious conflicts and repression, 154–158
  unprovoked denials, 146
de León, B., 32–35
delusions, 52–53
  "delusional metaphor," 62
denial, 174–176
  unprovoked denials, 146
"depression," 10–11
desire, 277–279
  analyst's, 121–122, 128
  in friendship dynamics, 108–109
  Graph of Desire, 224–225
  Other's desire, 197
  uncovering desire, 14
de Waal, F. B. M., 80, 91
"dialogue of the deaf," 36
"Direction of the Treatment" translation, 225–229. *See also* translation
disingenuous praise, 146. *See also* deception
displacement
  of affect, 158
  in psychotherapy, 167–169
divine love, 126
Dryden, J., 215

Écrits, 202
ED. *See* erectile dysfunction
Ekman, P., 83
Elisabeth Roudinesco's biography of *Jacques Lacan*, 285–288, 317
emotional ambivalence, 306
"enactments," 32
erectile dysfunction (ED), 174

erotomania, 306
"mortifying erotomania," 46
excuses, excessive, 145. *See also* deception
existential crisis, 63
existential-phenomenology, 242

Falzeder, E., 132
"family romance," 64
"father function." *See* "paternal function"
fears or phobias, 153
"feign feigning," 89–90
femme ondine symptôme (FOS), 134
Fink, B., 5, 16, 25, 31, 33, 103, 104, 120, 125, 222, 237
  exploring depths of psychoanalysis, 263–268
  Lacanian perspectives and clinical practice, 255–261
Flanders, S., 35–38
flawed thinkers, 272–273
fluency, 219. *See also* translation
"forced choice," 20
FOS. See *femme ondine symptôme*
Four Fundamental Concepts of Psychoanalysis, The, 260
frame, 305
French theory, 217–218. *See also* translation
Freudian slip, 149
Freud, S.
  affects, 9
  analysis of conflict and neurosis, 155–156
  analytic methods, 5
  anxiety, 10
  Clinical Introduction to Freud, A, 271–276
  concept of psychological defense, 151–154
  concepts and techniques, 276–276
  conscious and unconscious, 148–151
  countertransference and projection of responsibility, 114

emotional engagement, 127–128
evolution and psychoanalytic decision-making, 127
"family romance," 64
Freud-bashing, 272
hidden motives and betrayal, 143
intricacies of opposites, 147–148
Lacanian approach to, 255–261
later works, 257
limitations in psychoanalysis, 112–114
misjudgment in case of Dora, 112–114
"preliminary meetings," 25–26
psychical conflicts, 53
session length, 37
theory and practice, 5, 273–274, 275
transference, 41, 42
use of couch, 25
working with psychotics, 54
"full-blown paraphrenia," 62
fundamental fantasy, 193–196

gender transition, 307
Gherovici, P., 33, 249, 251
Graph of Desire, 224–225. *See also* translation
Grosskurth, P., 294
guilt, 11
  misalignment of, 167–169
  Rat Man's guilty affect, 111, 167–168

hate, transference, 110
hidden self and uninhibited expression, 145. *See also* deception
human gestures
  books about different, 85–86
  "feign feigning," 89–90
  human emotion interpretation, 84
  language and deceptive facade, 87
  role in human psychology, 79–80
  smiling, 81
  universality of facial gestures, 82–83

ideal ego, 20
imaginary, 77, 308. *See also* human gestures
   in animal behavior and human development, 77–79
   attraction in human beings, 79
   bared-teeth grin, 81–82
   deception and intentionality, 88
   dimension of human experience, 47
   as dyadic relations, 92–94
   ethology to psychoanalysis, 77–78
   "feign feigning," 89–90
   feigning and symbolism, 88–89
   illusion of altruism, 88
   imaginary register, 95–97
   as intuition, 98–99
   Knot theory, 98
   language and deceptive facade, 87
   meaning as, 97–98
   Other, 93
   overriding importance of images, 77–92
   register, 95–97
   role of images and body language, 79–80
   self-images and human ego, 79–80
   signifier and art of dissimulation, 89
   signs and social interactions, 91
   smiling in animal and human, 81
   symbolic behavior and number sense in animals, 91–92
   symbolism and psychosis, 94
   "think unnamed numbers," 92
   unambiguous emotional indicators, 86
   understanding as, 94
   universality of facial gestures, 82–83
   variability of human emotion interpretation, 84
interpersonal psychoanalysis. *See* relational psychoanalysis
intersubjectivity. *See* relational psychoanalysis

intuition, 98, 118
   conundrum of intuition and emotional responses, 120
   and countertransference, 8–9
   and subjectivity in psychoanalytic technique, 116–118

Jablonka, E., 78, 88
Jacques Lacan biography, 285–288, 317
Joseph, B., 309
jouissance, 49
   in psychoanalysis, 48–51
   psychotropic medications, 52
   real Other, 49
   symbolic Other, 49
   varied forms of, 48
"just because (I/we said so)" principle, 305

Kardiner, A., 113
Khoury, M., 33
Kleinian/Bionian psychoanalysis. *See* relational psychoanalysis
Knot theory, 98
Kuhn, T. S., 96

Lacanian psychoanalysis, 3, 303–305
   analyst-analysand relationship, 12–13
   analyst's role, 10–11, 12, 13
   analytic setting, 12, 25
   appeal among younger generations, 243–244
   "bedrock of castration," 17–18
   castration-oriented work, 21–22
   challenging assumptions, 23–24
   challenging roles, 12–13
   contrasting perspectives, 14–15
   countertransference, 7–9
   guilt in, 11
   influence of clinical and academic discourse, 244–245
   interpreting patient requests, 23
   Lacanian approach vs. contemporary views, 14–15

INDEX 331

Lacanian castration vs.
  conventional therapeutic
  gratification, 21–23
lack and loss, 17
Margulies on Lacanian theory and
  practice, 28–32
moroseness in, 11
neurosis, 35–38
neurotic and psychotic structures, 6
neurotic satisfaction, 16
paradox of ideology, 246–247
parental presence and analyst's
  interruptions, 15–16
reconciling Lacanian and
  non-Lacanian perspectives,
  32–35
responses to commentators, 27–38
rethinking affective states in, 10
role played by affects, 9–16
satisfaction, 16–17
scansion, 17–21, 27, 32, 35–38
separation, 16, 17
separation anxiety and aggressive
  wishes, 15–16
theory vs. practice, 246–247
treatment approaches to neurosis
  and psychosis, 6–7
unconscious expression in speech,
  7, 24–25
unconscious manifestations, 13
uncovering desire, 14
uniqueness and diversity in, 3–6
use of couch, 25–27
Lacan, J., 317
  biography of, 285–288
  challenging goal-oriented mindset,
    240
  depths of Lacanian thought, 237–254
  influence, 240
  Lacanian approach to Freud,
    255–261
  Lacan on Love, 125
  marginalization in academic and
    clinical psychology, 242–243
  perspectives, 249–250
  place in America, 238–239
  real, 307
  revival of Freudian thought,
    240–242
  rising interest in Lacan's work,
    239–240
  seminars, 319–320
  translators, 221–224
  transparent expression, 281–282
Lacan's works, translating, 201, 315.
  See also translation
  ambiguity in translating, 209–211
  challenges and misinterpretations
    in, 201, 224–230
  for clinicians, 213
  complexities of literary fidelity and
    interpretation, 215
  comprehensibility problems,
    209–211
  discrepancies and incoherences,
    205–207
  Écrits, 202
  interpreting polyvalent texts,
    209–211
  issues of source citation and
    context, 204–205
  linguistic errors and contextual
    ambiguities, 208–209
  problems with "establishment" of
    text, 202–209
  reconstructing meaning and
    misinterpretations, 207–208
  style problems, 211–215
  textual variation analysis, 203–204
lack and loss, 17
L'amour Lacan, 126
Lely, P., 105, 309
"Liar, The," 312–313
libidinal dynamics in psychosis, 45–47
Little, M., 37
loneliness, 251–252
Lorenz, C., 308
love, 14, 103, 308–310. *See also*
  deception
  analysts' desires for affection and
    recognition, 121–122
  analytic third, 118–119

and boundaries, 122
conundrum of intuition and emotional responses, 120
countertransference, 110
desires in friendship dynamics, 108–109
embracing lack in others, 106–108
embracing warts, 105–106
in flaws and fundamental differences, 105
Freud's countertransference and projection of responsibility, 114
Freud's limitations, 112–114
Freud's misjudgment in case of Dora, 112–114
and hate in dreams, 146
intuition and subjectivity, 116–118
and knowledge, 131–133
and nonexistence of sexual relationship, 135–139
"Other patient, the," 119
overidentification and erroneous conclusions, 112–114
paradox of analyst's role, 122
"patient's inner reality," 117
reframing countertransference, 115–116
relational psychoanalysis, 114–115
resistance in psychoanalysis, 111–112
impact of self-disclosure and analyst-driven dynamics, 120–121
shifting blame and virtue, 115–116
struggle with acceptance and clinical gaze, 106
transference, 104, 110, 305
unconscious and jouissance, 105
understanding love through lack and altruism, 109–110
use and abuse of countertransference, 110–122
love in Lacan's later work, 125, 310–311
analyst's emotional terrain, 128–130
Aristophanes' myth, 133–134
balancing flames of transference love, 126–127
crazy love, 133–135
divine love, 126
from divine to transference, 126
Freud's emotional engagement, 127–128
Freud's evolution and psychoanalytic decision-making, 127
getting something without really getting it, 131–133
love and nonexistence of sexual relationship, 135–139
love, belief, and skepticism in analytic relationship, 134–135
neutrality vs. smoldering, 126–131
obtaining the unobtainable, 131–133
paradox of giving and receiving, 133
paradox of love and knowledge, 131–133
philia, 136
subject-to-subject relationship, 137, 138
unconscious recognition, 137
"well-meaning neutrality," 128

Malan, D. H., 43, 66
Maleval, J.-C., 46, 47, 49, 51, 52, 54, 55, 59, 60, 62, 66, 67, 68, 70, 71, 282, 306, 307
Margulies, A., 28–32
megalomania, 62
melancholia, 61
"mental automatism," 60
mentorship, two faces of, 146–147. *See also* deception
Miller, J.-A., 287
Miller, M., 33
mirroring, 10
moral
   cowardice, 197
   failing, 11
moroseness, 11
"mortifying erotomania," 46

Name-of-the-Father, 259, 286
narcissism, 45
National Endowment for the
    Humanities (NEH), 239
NEH. See National Endowment for the
    Humanities
neurosis, 6, 35–38. See also neurotic(s)
    associations between parental
        figures and analyst, 69
    kind of Other in neurosis vs.
        psychosis, 66–69
    psychosis vs., 43–44
    transference characteristics in,
        42–45
    treatment approaches to, 6–7
neurotic(s), 306. See also psychotic(s)
    acting out, 48
    fundamental fantasy, 195
    Lacanian approach vs.
        contemporary views, 14–15
    neurotic's ego, 35
    neurotic's Other, 66–67
    obsessive, 55
    psychoanalytic setting in, 12
    psychotics vs., 31
    satisfaction, 16
    strategies for, 66–69
    structures, 6
    transference, 44–45

object-relation, 46
obsessive neurotics, 55
Ogden, T. H., 4, 114, 118, 119
ontological crisis, 63
opposites, 147–148
Ornstein, E., 294
"Other patient, the," 119
Other's desire, 197
Other, the, 93, 187
overidentification, 72, 112–114

"parapraxes." See "bungled actions"
"paternal function," 58
"paternal metaphor," 62–63
"patient's inner reality," 117
Peoc'h, M., 67, 282

philia, 136
phobias, 153
Pommier, G., 33
"preliminary meetings," 26
projection, 144, 309, 310. See also
    deception
psychical conflicts, 53
psychoanalysis, 155, 253
    challenges for, 248–249
    challenges of objectivity in, 119
    cross-pollination in American
        psychoanalytic schools,
        247–248
    disparity between theory and
        personal conduct, 272–273
    flawed thinkers, 272–273
    Freud's countertransference and
        projection of responsibility,
        114
    Freud's limitations, 112–114
    isolation and fear in modern
        society, 252–253
    jouissance in, 48–51
    loneliness, 251–252
    love and boundaries, 122
    outside mainstream, 254
    and politics, 245–246, 253–254
    psychoanalytic language, 282
    relational psychoanalysis, 114–115
    resistance, 111–112
    separation, 16
    shifting blame and virtue, 115–116
    theory and clinical practice,
        271–276
    transformative power of, 275–276
psychoanalytic language, 282
psychological defense mechanisms,
    151–154
psychosis, 6
    development and identification of
        psychotic structures, 70–71
    developmental stages of, 59–63
    kind of Other in neurosis vs.
        psychosis, 66–69
    libido dynamics in, 45–47
    neurosis vs., 43–44

ordinary, 65, 69–73
"sign of the mirror, the," 70
symbolism and, 94
therapeutic approaches, 6–7, 63–66
psychosis, ordinary, 65, 69
adapting identities, 71
adaptive strategies, 72–73
chameleon identities, 71–72
clinical signs and behavioral patterns, 73
development and identification of psychotic structures, 70–71
overidentification and ego, 72
psychotic(s), 278. *See also* neurotic(s)
historical perspectives on working with, 45–48
"as if" personality, 55
imaginary and real dynamics in, 47
needs and responses of, 48
vs. neurotics, 31
psychotic's Other, 66
strategies for, 66–69
structures, 6, 31
transference, 44–45
working with, 54–59

Rat Man's guilty affect, 111, 167–168
real, 307
real Other, 49
relational psychoanalysis, 114–115
Renik, O., 116, 117, 118, 310
repression, 143, 151–154. *See also* deception
consequences, 159
displaced feelings and suppressed emotions, 157–158
"displacement of affect," 158
example of, 154
schemas of, 158–162
unconscious conflicts and, 154–158
Roudinesco, E., 285–288, 317

satisfaction, 16–17
neurotic, 16
scansion, 17–21, 27, 32, 35–38
schizoid, 72
schizophrenia, 61
schizophrenic(s), 61
Schleiermacher, F., 216
Schreber, D. P., 58, 62, 70, 286, 306
self-disclosure, 120–121
self-images and human ego, 79–80
self-perception, 165–167, 312–315
"abandonment," 171–173
change in subjective position, 181–183
defiance and dependency, 178–180
diagnosis, 186–193
displacement in psychotherapy, 167–169
fundamental fantasy, 193–196
guilty pleasures, 180–181
intimacy and control, 174–175
labyrinth of deception, 169–171
misalignment of guilt, 167–169
Other's desire, 197
paradox of affection and denial in intimacy, 175–176
power of denial, 174–175
relationship to the Other, 187
from resistance to revelation, 183–185
rivalry, control, and, 176–178
seeking punishment, 178–180
transference, 183–185
unconscious, 196–197
unraveling fabrications in psyche, 169–171
Seminar VI, 277–279, 317
separation, 16, 17
anxiety, 15–16
setting, 305
sex-change operations, 307
"short sessions," 17
"sign of the mirror, the," 70
sliding signifiers, 232. *See also* translation
smiling, 81
Sokal, A., 217
Soler, C., 52, 137
source language, 218–219. *See also* translation
Spoto, D., 37
subject-supposed-to-know, 305

subject-to-subject relationship, 137, 138
submissive postures, 308
"Subversion of the Subject," 224. *See also* translation
supervision, 291, 317–318
    effective approaches in, 291–292
    factors influencing supervisee confidence, 292–293
    goals of, 292
    interpreting supervisee slips, 292
    Klein's perspective on supervision and countertransference, 294
    one-off supervision, 295
    principles and practices, 293
    self-disclosure, 294–295
Swales, S. S., 33, 143, 217
Sylvestre, M., 49, 50
symbolic Other, 49
systematic paraphrenia. *See* "full-blown paraphrenia"

target language, 219. *See also* translation
theoretical work translation, 218–220. *See also* translation
theory in translation, 224–230. *See also* translation
therapy veteran, 166
thinkers, flawed, 272–273
"think unnamed numbers," 92
Thorpe, W. H., 92
"thought disorder," 61
transference, 41, 183–185, 305–307
    in analytic practice, 45
    characteristics in neurosis, 42–45
    hate, 110
    historical perspectives on working with psychotics, 45–48
    imaginary and real dynamics in psychotic, 47
    jouissance in psychoanalysis, 48–51
    kind of Other in neurosis vs. psychosis, 66–69
    libidinal dynamics in psychosis, 45–47
    love, 104, 110, 126–127, 305
    needs and responses of psychotics in therapy, 48
    neurotics and psychotics, 44–45, 66–69
    object-relation, 46
    ordinary psychosis, 65, 69–73
    psychosis development stages, 59–66
    structure of psychotic difficulties, 53–54
    structuring psychotic experience, 51–52
    working with delusions, 52–53
    working with psychotics, 54–59
"transitivism," 24
translation, 217, 219, 316. *See also* Lacan's works, translating
    challenge of translating "Direction of the Treatment," 225–229
    challenges and responsibilities, 231–234
    challenges in translating theoretical works, 218–220
    distinction between exposing and facilitating insight, 233–234
    distortion of French theory, 217–218
    errors in understanding French, 230–231
    impact of flawed, 229–230
    fluency, 219
    "foolish undertaking" and/or "thankless task," 215–216
    Graph of Desire, 224–225
    importance of accurate, 233
    Lacan's translators, 221–224
    mistranslations of Lacan's work, 220–224
    production of, 218–220
    significance and limits of sliding signifiers, 232
    source language, 218–219
    "Subversion of the Subject," 224
    target language, 219
    theory in, 224–230
Tyack, P. L., 80, 91

unconscious, 148–151, 196–197
	conflicts and repression, 154–158
	deciphering, 306
	desires in friendship dynamics, 108–109
	expression in speech, 7, 24–25
	manifestations, 13
	recognition, 137
uninhibited expression and hidden self, 145. *See also* deception
unprovoked denials, 146

Weinstein, L., 294
"well-meaning neutrality," 128
Whitaker, R., 183, 314
Winer, J., 294
Winnicott, D. W., 12, 24, 34, 37, 307

www.ingramcontent.com/pod-product-compliance
Ingram Content Group UK Ltd.
Pitfield, Milton Keynes, MK11 3LW, UK
UKHW021614220126
467229UK00012B/332